shortcuts to
sexy
abs

shortcuts to
sexy abs

COLLEEN MORIARTY

337 Ways to Trim, Tone, Camouflage and Beautify

APPLE

Published in the UK in 2004 by
Apple Press
Sheridan House
112-116A Western Road
Hove
East Sussex BN3 1DD
England
www.apple-press.com

10 9 8 7 6 5 4 3 2 1

ISBN 1-84092-455-1

Cover and book design by Laura McFadden Design, Inc.
Laura.mcfadden@rcn.com

Printed and bound in Canada

The information in this book is for educational purposes only.
It is not intended to replace the advice of a physician or medical practitioner.
Please see your health care provider before beginning any new health program.

*To Jeffery S. Weston, my loving husband and best
friend who is always by my side through it all, and to our
daughter, Bliss Ashlynn Weston, for whom I happily sacrificed
my abs to bring into this world and who has filled my
life with belly laughs ever since.*

[contents]

Foreword   8

Introduction   15

Chapter 1

The Great Date Plan   **22**
~ *Health and Beauty Bytes*   24
~ *Fitness Fun*   30
~ *Nutrition Nuggets*   40
~ *Fashion Facts*   51
~ *The Cardio Workout*   58

Chapter 2

**The Look Marvelous
at the Office Plan**   **64**
~ *Health and Beauty Bytes*   66
~ *Fitness Fun*   71
~ *Nutrition Nuggets*   82
~ *Fashion Facts*   94
~ *The Yoga Workout*   103

Chapter 3

The Fabulous Party Plan 110

~ *Health and Beauty Bytes* 112
~ *Fitness Fun* 120
~ *Nutrition Nuggets* 132
~ *Fashion Facts* 143
~ *10-Minute Cardio Workouts* 153

Chapter 4

**The Get Your Abs Back
After Pregnancy Plan** 164

~ *Health and Beauty Bytes* 167
~ *Fitness Fun* 179
~ *Nutrition Nuggets* 188
~ *Fashion Facts* 196
~ *Post-Pregnancy Waistline
Whittling Exercises* 202

Chapter 5

The Bikini Beach Plan 208

~ *Health and Beauty Bytes* 210
~ *Fitness Fun* 245
~ *Nutrition Nuggets* 247
~ *The Look Great in a Bikini Workout* 252

Acknowledgments 255

About the Author 256

The Ab Fad

I'm not a slacker. It's just that I'm always looking for a shortcut, a quicker route, expediency, a way to save time and cheat the system a little. I'm the person who reads and tries every workout article that promises it'll all be over in five minutes or less. Because, come on, who really wants to do more when you can do less? And truth be told, I'm trying to rush through that five-minute workout to make it four. That's why when I started noticing waistbands in the fashion magazines doing the limbo—dipping lower below the belly button than ever before—I hoped it was just a fad that would go away. But it didn't. Clothes just kept getting skimpier, with low-rise jeans now hovering as low as three inches below the navel and cute midriff-peeking tops riding upwards. Like it or not, abs have become the fitness and beauty obsession du jour: longer, leaner, sleeker, sexier, trimmer, and tighter. What was I to do? Yeah, I'm thin enough at a size four post-baby, but long ago I realized I'd never achieve a six pack stomach without taking up residence at the health club, so I embraced my softer middle. But with this new belly-baring trend, unless I wanted to start shopping stores that catered to mature, button-up, great-grandmother types, I had to find a way to get the latest fashion and beauty accessory (phenomenal abdominals) without having to spend my life at the gym.

As a beauty, health, and fitness writer, this ab obsession was one trend I just couldn't ignore. Glance at any magazine, music video, or celebrity donning clingy clothes on the red carpet and it's clear the abs have emerged as the anatomical feature of the moment. Even if you're thinking yours are a long way off from being ready to bare to the world, rest easy. (But that doesn't mean showing off a jelly belly like lots of women are these days.) It is possible to take those abs from flab to fab—and unlike other abs of steel, sculpted abs, or killer ab books out there, you won't have to quit your job and say good-bye to the kids, husband, or boyfriend for six months while you try to train away that Pooh belly. There are plenty of quick and easy ways (thank heavens) to minimize your middle and get the abs of the moment—or at least fake it—no matter how much or how little time you have on your hands. Only got a minute, ten minutes, thirty minutes? Easy and breezy beauty, fitness, and nutrition fixes can help. Got more time? Explore other fun ways to get celebrity abs without having to stop eating, live at a gym, or re-mortgage your home to hire a personal trainer and plastic surgeon.

With the fashion and fitness focus shifted away from genetically engineered areas like breasts and legs, there's a fairness to this latest body craze. Anyone can work toward more amazing abs. That's not true when it comes to being voluptuous or having mile-high legs. No matter how hard I try, I just can't gain two cup sizes or grow longer gams. Not only that, but the exercises that make the tummy totally toned don't require a gym membership. They can largely be done at home with no, or relatively little, equipment. So, in a lot of ways, this body craze is for the masses. Anyone, anywhere, anytime can work toward a celebrity-sexy stomach. The other good news is that the hard body, six-pack stomach and abs of steel are as passé as stirrup pants—a relief if you had resigned yourself to the fact that you couldn't "make it burn" long enough to even have a three pack. The abs of the moment are athletic, taut, and toned, but elongated. Today it's about getting a longer, leaner line.

So get ready to let your belly peek out of a flirty, cropped top!

At the core

Even though belly exposure is in vogue, flattening out your abs shouldn't be your only motivation for getting a marvelous middle. Your abs, along with your back muscles, are your body's support structure. Your abs and back muscles make up what fitness experts now call your core. These core muscles provide your body its deep-down strength—giving your body the scaffolding it needs to stand tall, lift heavy objects (like a box or a toddler), and look totally toned in whatever you wear—or in nothing at all. A strong core also helps prevent back pain and gives you the freedom to enjoy your favorite sports and everyday activities. So, unlike other frivolous fashion accessories, your abs really can be both functional and fabulous.

What is the core? The core consists of your ab and back muscles. There are four main muscle groups that make up the abdominals. They are:

1. The rectus abdominis

The rectus abdominis runs vertically to the pelvis from the lower ribs. It is a long, flat muscle spanning the front of the abdomen. These muscles control forward bending (spinal flexation). This is the muscle people mistakenly refer to as the "upper" and "lower" abs. In fact, it's all one muscle, the rectus abdominis. Some exercises will work more of the upper or lower portion of the muscle, but you cannot choose to train one or the other exclusively, as it's one muscle, not two.

2. The external oblique

Connected to the rectus abdominis are the external obliques, which run diagonally downward from the lower ribs to the pelvis. These broad, thin muscles help bend the spine from side to side (spinal flexation) and are therefore the muscles to tone when you want slimmer sides.

3. The internal oblique

These muscles lie below the external obliques and are smaller and thinner than their external siblings. They curve upwards to the lower ribs and also are recruited for rotation.

4. The transversus abdominis

The transverse abdominis concentrates in the bikini area. This deep vertical muscle contracts when the other three are working and can't be targeted by itself in your workout, but it is tightened and toned when you work your other abdominal muscles. It holds your internal organs in place, supports your spine, and is activated during breathing.

While it's not important for you to have a deep understanding of the intricacies of the ab anatomy, it is important to have a general grasp of which muscles you are targeting when working toward a sexier midsection. Exercise physiologists and mind/body experts say it's always a good idea for you to visualize what muscle you want to engage before executing each move. Take a second to mentally practice each exercise before doing it, picturing which muscles are involved (i.e., doing side twists will engage the obliques). This will help your form and make sure you are contracting the right muscle, making your ab exercises more effective.

Shortcuts to Sexy Abs: 337 Ways to Trim, Tone, Camouflage, and Beautify isn't just chock full of easy exercises to achieve a sleeker tummy. Unlike other ab books out there, this book also focuses on easy ways to complement your workout efforts—using health, nutrition, beauty, and fashion tips from experts I've interviewed over the last eight years—to make your middle look longer, leaner, thinner, and sexier. ~

[introduction]

Think about abs, and two images come to mind. First, you think about red carpet abs—the sleek and sexy stomachs of starlets parading down the red carpet at the Oscars with flashes popping snapshots of their unabashedly exposed bellies. Then your mind also conjures images of the six-pack, body builder stomach. If you compare these two images, you can see how vastly different the looks are. The first appears the product of perfect genes. The second looks like it's the product of a lot of hard work. The latter is true of both. Having a hardbody, six-pack stomach does take lots of dedication and hard work. But so does the more updated long, lean, and limber look that so many celebrities are sporting right now and we're all hoping to achieve. According to the Hollywood personal trainers I've spoken to, these starlets weren't born with totally toned tummies. They work at them—with targeted ab exercises, yoga, Pilates, good nutrition, cardio workouts, and beauty fixes. This book reveals the tricks and training secrets for Oscar-worthy abs.

When I started becoming obsessed with abs, I was like many people. I was thin enough and looked good in clothes, but my sides were pinchable after eight years of marriage. My paunch was poochy even after losing all the baby weight from having my daughter. The skin was loose and jiggly, especially around the belly button. I looked good enough—as long as my husband loved me the way I was—because no one else was going to see me anyway. That was until navel-showing clothing because so popular and all of a sudden jeans that covered the belly button were frumpy. Suddenly, having a sexy stomach really mattered if I wanted to look good in the latest fashions. Over the course of a year, I started exercising more faithfully—walking, jogging, doing yoga videos, hiking, and biking. And I started pitching more story ideas that required me to talk to personal trainers, physical therapists, nutritionists, and beauty pros about how in the world you could get a sexier stomach. My conclusion after speaking to my Rolodex of experts—without whom this book would never have been written—was that having amazing abs wasn't out of reach. I really could get my pre-pregnancy body back, plus work toward losing those love handles and making my middle younger and more toned looking. I was also surprised at how simple their advice was. These were tips I could really follow—that anybody could incorporate into her life.

My middle became more toned and I eventually got up the courage to buy extra-low slung jeans (which, by the way, are also a whole lot more comfortable than ones that rise above the navel). But another surprising benefit awaited me. I had been weak in my core abdominal muscles after having a c-section. I'd felt like my power-house strength was lost forever. Having a toddler who loved riding on my hip was wonderful until she started to become so heavy that my back would sing with pain whenever I picked her up. I'd never in my life suffered any back trouble and I couldn't believe how disabling and scary it was to want to lie flat on my back and not move—let alone take care of my baby. Just walking, sitting, or turning my neck could be excruciating. I was sure a chiropractor or orthopedic surgeon was in my future. But doing the core training to get my abs in shape also strengthened my back; I was again able to lift heavy objects and enjoy my everyday activities pain free. I could carry my best girl around a store, tickle her upside down, pick her up easily—and heft a diaper bag too. I felt more confident and in control, and my posture improved too, giving me an uplifted and slimmer appearance.

As a beauty writer, I also wanted to address the not-so-flattering effects of having a baby and a C-section: stretch marks, loose skin, and jelly belly. And, of course, there are things women in general have to contend with: loss of muscle tone, a widening middle, and, to some extent, sagging skin. All the answers I found to these nagging problems are here in this book.

How to use this book

You can read this book from start to finish, but I figure most women start to get bugged by their abs when they are thinking about a specific event (such as a hot date or a Valentine's Day party). Therefore, I've created specific plans for the various times you'll want to look and feel your best, including that special date, looking great at the office, going to a fabulous party, getting your abs back after pregnancy, and strolling down the beach in an incredibly sexy bikini.

Each chapter contains Health and Beauty Bytes, Fitness Fun, Nutrition Nuggets, and Fashion Facts. If you're pregnant or have just had a baby, you'll find advice and tips for during and post-pregnancy to care for your abs so that, sooner rather than later, no matter what your present condition, your abs will be as flat and as sexy as you want. Finally, at the end of each chapter, I've included a workout program that will help you build great abs and keep them!

There is one overall guiding principle of this book: Magic fast fixes do exist. It's not too late to get a more bare-able belly tonight. Tap into these fast nutrition, beauty, and fashion tips that really can make your abs look more amazing. But, for lasting results and to make a real change it takes:

workbook

While it is impossible to spot-reduce (you can't only exercise for your abs and expect the weight to come off from there and not anywhere else), it is possible to create realistic exercise routines that target certain goals. The workouts in this book are specific to each chapter's goal.

• **Cardio for your sexy dates.** These exercise plans will help you burn fat and calories to drop a size or two, thus making your torso (and everything else) smaller.

• **Yoga for killer abs at the office.** Your stress level has been shown to be directly related to the amount of fat you carry around your middle. Yoga will not only tone and strengthen your abs and back muscles, it will also help you relax and renew and lose that stress-related excess. You'll be calm and gorgeous!

1) Exercise to truly tone your tummy, 2) a healthy diet to prevent gaining belly fat and to help fuel you through your workouts and your everyday activities, and 3) cardiovascular workouts to help burn existing fat. The 337 simple shortcuts in this book can help to get your midsection shaped up for tonight and the rest of your life! ~

- **Ten-minute workouts for the fabulous party plan.** I don't expect you to drop and give me ten right in front of the buffet table, but studies have shown that short bursts of intense exercise (ten minutes worth) are an effective way to remain fit. The key is making them intense (brisk walks instead of strolls, for example) and doing at least three of them every day.
- **Want to whittle your waist after the baby?** My post-baby workout focuses on the obliques—the muscles that run from your back to your front and, when tight and toned, create the indentation of your waist.
- **Pilates for a bikini body.** You've never worn a bikini? Well, you will come summer. Pilates exercises create long, lean muscles and flat, fabulous abs. These are the moves of ballerinas—and no one has flatter bellies than ballet dancers. You'll be amazed how, in just a few sessions, you'll stand taller and look leaner.

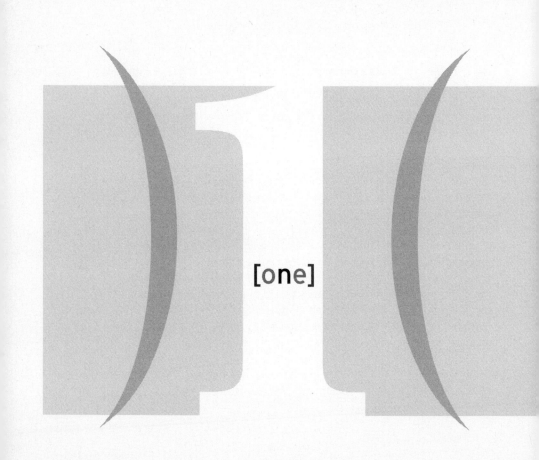

[one]

The Great Date Plan

Whether it's a first date, the all-important third date, the night you think he'll propose, or even a celebration of 20 years together, nothing feels better than knowing your man thinks you look hot! And, for most men, a small waist-to-hip ratio is like a dish of milk to a kitty-cat—nothing attracts a man like a curvy torso. The good news is that women of all shapes and sizes can have (or just look like they have) the perfect hourglass figure.

In this chapter, you'll find tips on dressing sexy, finding clothes that have a certain va-va-va-voom, changing the way you eat to reduce bloating, and exercising to burn off extra fat and calories. By the time your date rolls around, you'll be able to strut your stuff feeling sexy and feminine.~

Health and Beauty Bytes

)1(Use a body scrub

As any scrubaholic will tell you, using a body polish scrubs away dead skin cells for a smoother-looking stomach. Incorporate a quick, 60-second tummy polish into your shower a couple times a week to eliminate dead skin cells and make your stomach look smoother and sleeker.

)2(Take a sauna

A steambath or sauna promotes sweating which helps your body flush out excess water and toxins. Using a dry brush on your skin before getting into the heat will bring a healthy glow to your skin and will encourage better circulation.

)3(Look five pounds thinner with makeup

To look trimmer, avoid highlighting your cheeks with blush, which creates fullness. Instead, accentuate your eyes for a thinner look. Try a nude palette of browns, tans, and taupes. Use the lightest buff color all over from eye to brow. Then use a sweep of the medium shade on the outer corners of your eye bone. Try outlining your eyes with a damp eye shadow brush instead of eyeliner. Choose a dark espresso shade. Draw even more attention to your eyes with strokes of mascara on the upper, outer corners of your eyelashes.

)4(Dab on a slimming scent

Wear a floral-and-spice fragrance and the world may instantly see you as slimmer. Researchers at the Smell and Taste Treatment and Research Foundation in Chicago had 199 men inhale fragrances then guess how much the women who wore them weighed. Spicy-floral blends scored lower numbers—meaning the women were perceived to weigh an average of 12 pounds less than their actual weight.

)5(Get checked for slimming saboteurs

Belly fat may signal an undiagnosed health problem. Such problems can include depression, which can increase eating and weight gain and reduce ability to sleep, which can then compound the weight gain and exacerbate emotional problems. Polycystic Ovary Syndrome is another condition that affects about three percent of women. The body overproduces the hormone androgen, leading to problems such as weight gain, acne, irregular periods, infertility, and abnormal hair growth. When diagnosed, doctors can prescribe medication to control hormone production. Conditions such as Irritable Bowel Syndrome can cause abdominal bloating, so see your doctor to rule out any health complications.

)6(Talk to your doctor

Contrary to popular lore, if your scale won't budge except in the wrong direction, the birth control pill probably isn't to blame. In a recent study, nearly fifty percent of women were under the opinion that the Pill causes weight gain. In another study, three placebo-controlled randomized trials did not find evidence that the Pill (oral or skin patch) causes weight gain. But some drugs are pound-promoting:

- Depo-Provera birth control shot
- Antidepressants (Elavil or lithium for bipolar disorder)
- Other psychiatry drugs are associated with weight gain in as many as forty percent of patients, according to experts.

)7(Spit out your gum

Chewing gum for too long, especially sugarless gum, causes you to gulp excess air that can bloat your middle. And it's a crummy habit to bring on a date—no one can kiss someone who's chewing gum! If you want to chew gum to clean your teeth (it does work!) or freshen your breath (ditto!) then chew until you feel it has taken effect, then take it out to avoid getting too much gas in your belly.

)8(Ask your doctor about the Yasmin birth control pill

It contains a unique form of progestin that is based on a diuretic which will help prevent water weight gain. Your doc may also recommend the diuretic hydrochlorothiazide (HCTZ). Given in low doses during the last two weeks of the cycle, this product can help solve monthly swelling.

Fitness Fun

)9(Sit properly

Sitting properly makes you look taller and more relaxed. And sitting upright allows food to settle in the lower part of your stomach, helping you feel satiated and less likely to want a second serving. Good posture at the table starts at your butt. Make sure both cheeks sit evenly on the chair. Your feet should both be on the floor, or crossed at your ankles. Keep your pelvis in neutral—just like when you're standing—and make sure your shoulders are relaxed and even. Your chin should be parallel to the floor or tilted slightly down.

)10(Give the mouse a house

Here's a fabulous exercise for a flatter lower belly. Lie on your back, knees bent, feet on the floor, arms along your sides. On an inhale, bring your belly button in toward your spine and flatten your back against the floor. Then, exhale slowly and let your back curve up (making a house for a mouse on the floor under you). Do this move very slowly with deep breaths up to 10 times per day.

)11(Beat the bloat

Does PMS make you feel like a beached whale? Research from the Journal of Psychosomatic Obstetrics and Gynecology shows that massage therapy not only reduces premenstrual anxiety, depressed moods, and discomfort, it also reduces water retention, which is good news for flattening your tummy during that time of the month.

)12(Weighted crunches

Lie on your back with your feet flat on the floor, knees bent. Clasp a small dumbbell in your hands and hug it to your chest. Contract your abs and slowly raise your head, neck, and shoulders off the floor. Keep your belly button pulled into your spine. Hold. Gently lower yourself back down to the starting position. Do two sets of 8 to 15 reps. Increase the weight over time as this move becomes easy. If you have back problems or feel any strain in your lower back, skip the weights.

)13(Towel toners

Spread out a bath towel and lie down on your back with your head along the top edge. Hold the corners of the towel with each hand, knees bent and feet flat on the floor. Inhale and pull your belly button in toward your spine. Exhale and contract your abs and lift your head, neck, and shoulders off the floor with the towel. Stay in this position. Inhale and slide your right heel forward along the floor until your leg is fully extended. Exhale and bring the leg back, drawing your foot along the floor to the starting position. Alternate legs and do 15 to 20 reps.

) 14 (Always wear a sports bra

Nothing makes boobs sag like lots of jumping and running. When you try on a sports bra, jump around in the dressing room to see how much bounce you get. The less movement, the better, for your comfort and for keeping gravity from drawing everything southbound. Perky breasts make the middle look slimmer.

workbook

)15(Swivel and Swirl your Way to Slimmer Sides

When you think of belly dancing, coined belts, undulating pelvises, and sideways shaking hips probably come to mind. Belly dancing is also a hot aerobic workout. What's alluring about belly dancing is that it raises your heart rate for a cardio workout, trims and tones your middle, and makes you feel you can charm with your hips, not just your personality!

Here are three belly dancing moves to do on your own. Try them in a sequence:

1. Stomach pulses Stand on a 45-degree angle, legs together, hands resting on the sides of your head above your ears. Pulse your stomach in and out. Repeat five times each side twice.

2. Belly dance toe taps Step to the right then tap the ground with your left toe. Now step to the left and tap your right toe. Keep going, adding in this arm motion: As you step to the right, extend your right arm out to the side from your elbow and raise your left arm over your left ear and sway toward the right. Switch arms as you toe tap to the left. Meanwhile, pulse your abs in and out each time your toe taps down.

3. Pelvic thrusts Stand again at a 45-degree angle with your legs together, this time with your hands resting on your hips. Pulse your pelvis and abs in and out. Do this five times on each side. Repeat. Go back to belly dance toe taps.

For more on belly dancing, call your local gym or dance studio to see if they offer a belly dancing class. Or check out a wide variety of fitness-oriented belly dancing videos to try at home.

)16(Belly bulge busters

Lie on your back, right knee bent, foot flat on the floor. Bend your left leg and put your left foot squarely on a small ball. Tighten your abs and roll the ball away from you until your left leg is extended. Roll back to starting position. Do one set of 12 to 15 reps. Switch sides and repeat.

)17(Turn off the boob tube

TV is okay for a short time (say thirty minutes to an hour at most), but anything longer than that will increase your stress level and decrease your metabolism. If you find yourself searching for something to watch with the remote control, do something else! If you are watching TV, at least get up during the commercials or, if you can, consider using the commercial time to fit in a set of ab exercises or even some spins with the jump rope.

)18(Bent-knee curl ups

Lie on your back with your knees bent and feet flat on the floor. Keep your heels twelve to eighteen inches from your buttocks. Fold your arms across your chest and place your palms on opposite shoulders. Contract your abs and gently and slowly curl upwards, raising your back and shoulder blades off the floor while pressing your belly button toward your spine and your low back into the floor. Slowly roll back down. Do one to two sets of 15 reps.

)19(Workout Kellys

This move is named after the girl in my college gym who introduced me to this move and had the most amazing abs on campus. If you belong to a gym, try this move on a bench. If not, clear your coffee table and pad it with a towel or mat. Lie on your back where you can reach over your head and hold the edge of the bench or table behind you with your elbows bent and close to your ears. Bend your knees and raise them so that your knees are directly over your hips and your knees and feet are together and parallel to the ground. Tighten your ab muscles and gently move your bent knees a few inches toward your chest so that your buttocks and pelvis are a few inches off the bench or table. Pulse legs upwards for 10 counts and lower. Repeat. Work up to two sets of 8 to 12 reps.

)20(Exercise like a kid

Children have an innate way of being active—they go all out for a few minutes, then collapse, then get their energy back and go all out again, then collapse. While I don't recommend collapsing, you should try to get some all-out intense minutes of exercise on most days of the week. You can't keep that energy expenditure going for too long (which is why kids naturally stop moving that hard) but getting your heart rate up that much is good for your health and your waistline.

)21(Have a mini-meal

Going out tonight? Have a mini-meal before your date. Eating a small and healthy meal ensures that you won't overindulge when you finally sit down for that candlelight dinner, packing yourself full of excess calories and fat. Not only will downing superhero-sized restaurant portions make you feel like you're going to pop a button on those low-slung jeans, but overeating causes gas and bloating in the abdomen. Try a chunk of lean turkey and low-fat cheese dipped in mustard or veggie sticks (peppers, carrots, and celery) dipped in fat-free dressing to hold you over.

)22(Watch your fruit intake

Fruits can be a source of intestinal bloating and gas. Excess fructose can remain in the large intestine, where it ferments and causes gas. This is what makes you feel swollen. Some fruits and juices contain a lot of fructose: apples, apricots, cherries, pears, plums, prunes, and peaches. On a day when you want to flatten your abs, limit your portions of these foods as well as processed foods that contain high-fructose corn sweeteners. Read labels to figure out which foods contain them—the closer the words "high-fructose corn syrup" appear to the top of the ingredient list, the more the product contains. Look for this especially on breads, crackers, and juices.

)23(Learn your portion sizes

Most women need to eat meals that are the size of two fists together, while a snack is the size of one fist (or what can fit in your palm, such as seven almonds). Anything above that and your stomach will be forced to expand!!

)24(Choose one treat at a restaurant

Decide if your caloric splurge is going to be bread, wine, or dessert—then stick to that at the restaurant. One splurge per customer!

workbook

)25(Did you know?

Bartenders push peanuts, pretzels, and Chex Mix because when you pop salty foods into your mouth, you'll get thirsty quicker and more often, so you'll order more drinks. Not only will the salty foods add to your bar tab, they'll add excess calories. The alcohol can also cause a bloated look the next morning. Ask the bartender to take these snacks away so the bottomless bowl isn't refilled over and over. Other restaurant foods to beware of that contain high amounts of sodium:

- Margaritas
- Salsa
- Pizza
- Cream sauces
- Soups

)26(Order wine

When ordering a drink, opt for wine instead of beer or spirits. Both are correlated with higher waist circumference (that means a meatier middle) later in life for those who slosh it back regularly. Wine drinkers, however, have smaller waists. But, before you say, "Another Merlot, please!" recognize that wine is an appetite stimulant and source of calories. So for a sexy stomach, sip sparingly.

)27(Close your mouth

Talking while you eat is not only rude, it'll cause your tummy to fill up with excess air. It's easy to be nervous on a date (I always was!), but if you focus on remaining calm and chewing your food, you'll actually settle your nerves and keep you belly flat and beautiful.

)28(Choose these fast foods (if you must)

At a Mexican joint? Go vegetarian and hold the refried beans. Choose black beans with rice, plenty of lettuce, and go easy on the full-fat cheese, sour cream, and tortillas. (No chips!)

Burgers? Eat the kids' meal (you'll get a prize!) which will save you calories and let you enjoy a complete meal. Or, cut down on anything with dressing or anything that's fried. Pile on the vegetables and enjoy any salad they offer (but use the salad dressing sparingly).

Chicken? A grilled sandwich is usually safe. Try to add some vegetables to round out the meal. You can always eat the meat and skip the roll to reduce the amount of carbs and calories.

)29(Sniff your food

Like sniffing a fine wine, smell your food before delving into your meal. The olfactory glands help release a satiety hormone that makes you feel fuller faster, so you can eat less and feel satisfied sooner.

)30(Think oil, not butter

Dipping your bread (whole grain is best) in olive oil, rather than spreading it with butter, can save you calories and make your heart healthier. The fats in olive oil are better for you than those in butter.

)31(Cut your portion in half

Almost sixty percent of women finish their restaurant portion, even though most of those women also say they are served too much food. Ask for appetizers, rather than entrées as your main course or simply split your entrée in half as soon as its served and bring the rest home to enjoy tomorrow.

)32(It's the sauce that counts

Often what makes a great meal great isn't the added fat (after all, you can cook something in olive oil or butter), but the fabulous sauces and reductions. If you're at a fine restaurant, look for dishes that are broiled or sautéed in wine and stay away from anything breaded or fried.

)33(Don't create a disorder

Some people try to keep their stomach from pooching out by cleaning out their intestines with laxatives. This is usually not a good idea. These measures should only be taken if recommended by a doctor. Otherwise, your food may pass through your system faster than vitamins, nutrients, and minerals can be absorbed by the body, robbing you of vital nutrition. Some laxatives may also contribute to dehydration by removing fluids.

)34(Eat protein at every meal

Protein helps you feel full and staves off blood sugar spikes, which make your energy (and hunger) levels fluctuate. Some good protein snacks include string cheese, peanut butter, nuts, hard cheese, lunch meat, and hard-boiled eggs.

)35(Get your thyroid checked

If your thyroid isn't working properly, your metabolic rate can drop. That means your metabolism and fat-burning rate can slow down significantly. Ask your doctor if your thyroid could be contributing to a weight problem.

)36(Start your day with hot lemonade

The yogis I know swear by this trick. Heat four cups of water. As you're doing that, squeeze the juice of one lemon into a quart container. Add a tablespoon or so of honey. Pour the water over this mixture, stir, and drink (but not all at once, try a glass every hour). This is a natural diuretic that will help fight fluid retention.

)37(Never say diet

Dieting does not have long term success for most people, and it often involves reducing your food intake, calories, and food variety to unhealthy levels. Many fad diets require you to cut out entire food groups, which isn't wise. Instead, eat a wide variety of foods rather than depriving yourself. But do eliminate the big offenders that are nutritionally void and deliver a lot of fat, carbohydrates, and calories: soda, chips, junk food, fried foods, and desserts. Also, on days when your abs need to look their best, eat a low- or no-carb diet. Certainly don't eliminate carbs from your diet altogether without the advice of your doctor or nutritionist. When you do eat carbs, keep them to a minimum (one slice of bread instead of two) and stick to whole grain products only.

Fashion Facts

)38(**Bring his eye elsewhere**

All important third date? If you're feeling self-conscious about your waist, make sure he's looking somewhere else—your eyes, your hair, your décolletage, your legs. You'll feel more confident and he'll be smitten! The key to playing up one particular feature is to be dramatic— use eye-liner, tousle your hair, wear a low-cut blouse or a daring mini-skirt. You can control where his eyes go! Also, by reminding yourself that you have many more beautiful qualities than just your belt size, you'll feel better about yourself, too.

)39(**Wear a corset**

Think I'm kidding? A small waist-to-hip ratio is what's sexiest to many a man. To find out what your ratio is, divide your waist circumference by your hip circumference—such as 32 divided by 41. You're looking for a number between 0.6 and 0.7. If you're not there yet, consider a corset (these days they're made of lycra, not whale stays), which will whittle your waist in minutes.

)40(**Try fringe**

Dresses or blouses with fringe will bring the eyes of others to your clothes, rather than your belly. Whether it's on the arms, hems, or all over the dress like the flappers in the 1920s, you'll look fun, festive, and fabulous.

)41(Slip on some heels

Just a 1.5-inch heel helps you carry yourself taller, making you look leaner. Heels also make your legs look longer and leaner. If you have trouble walking in heels, try the stacked versions, which are wider. However, nothing slims a body like a pair of stilettos! If you have lower back problems, avoid heels and stick to other shortcuts, especially the core strengtheners.

)42(Try an Empire waist

Tops or dresses with a high empire waist (the waist line comes to a point just under and between your breasts) direct the eye up and away from your middle for a slimmer look. Empire (pronounced "am-peer") waistlines also give the illusion of a fuller and perkier bust.

)43(Tie on a belt

Try a fashion-forward tie-belt, worn diagonally and sitting slightly lower on one hip. Creating a diagonal line (rather than horizontal) is a TV trick to make your waist look smaller.

)44(Go for boy-cut

Underwear that hits just below, or just above, the fullest part of your middle is most flattering. Bikini strings that "cut into" the tummy will make it look bumpier.

)45(Top it off

Choose a top with detailing at the neck to draw the eye up and away from the trouble zone. Laces, embroidery, or a contrasting color all work to bring attention to that part of the blouse or dress.

)46(Necklaces can steal the show

A really nice necklace—the more unusual and proportional to your shape the better—can bring all the attention upwards and away from your midsection. What does proportional to your shape mean? If you're a small woman (5'4" and under), keep the jewelry more delicate than if you're tall and big-boned. Tall and small-boned? Delicate works best for you, too.

) 47 (Never wear faded denim

Deep, dark denim is most slimming and will make you look like you dropped five pounds. Go for bootcut legs—the slightly flared ankle area makes your tummy, hips, and butt look smaller in comparison to a wider leg versus a skinny, pencil pant leg. This style makes sure your middle isn't the widest surface of your pants.

) 48 (Highlight your best feature

Choose a bright color or pattern for your slimmest feature and basic black or charcoal for everywhere else. The dark colors help hide a lot, and by carefully placing your color you'll control where you want the eye to go.

)49(Think below-the-waist

If you need to slim your abs immediately, avoid tops that hit you at the waist. Look through your closet for a shirt or jacket that is slightly longer, hitting ideally at the hip bone or mid-butt.

)50(Slip on low-rise jeans

Jeans and pants that sit just below your navel make your torso look longer, making you look taller and slimmer.

The Cardio Workout

Here are three cardio routines. Feel free to mix and match these programs. Each one burns fat and calories, creating a sleek and slimmer body (all of it, not just your abs!).

These plans can be used with a heart-pumping activity (walking or running, swimming, biking, the elliptical trainer, or the Stair Master). Aim for 30 minutes for each cardio session and, remember, mixing up your workouts (walking one day and swimming the next) challenges your heart and muscles more than staying with one activity every day.

)51(Interval

Walk at 3.5 mph for five minutes. Increase the speed to 6 mph for two minutes. Come back down to 4 mph for three minutes. Alternate between the two speeds three more times (until 25 minutes are up) then go back down to 3.5 mph for the last five minutes.

)52(Pyramid

Walk at 3.5 mph for five minutes. Every two minutes increase your speed by a .5 mph so that you end up at 6 mph, which is a run. Come back down by a .5 mph every two minutes. Walk at 3.5 mph for the last five minutes to cool down.

)53(Intensify your workout

Instead of tacking on extra minutes to your cardio workout, try intensifying your workout. You can burn more calories in less time by working out more intensely. One way to do that is with interval training. Vary your speed when jogging—walk for a couple minutes, then jog, then run. The distance between two phone poles is a favorite meter for when you should shift gears and speed. You'll get your heart rate up and boost your metabolism to continue burning calories after the workout as well.

)54(Stroll

One day a week (at least) don't worry about intensity and, instead, worry about enjoyment! Research shows a 30-minute walk five days a week whittles the middle. Walkers lose twice as much belly fat as dieters. In one study scientists found a stroll a day is all it takes to get that jelly belly to go away and stay at bay for good. One group of women was asked to walk 30 minutes per day. The control group was asked to diet. After 12 weeks, the walkers walked away with bikini-worthy abs. Walkers also scored by reducing artery-clogging cholesterol levels. Regular walks help melt away flab along with stress—so you'll look and feel more streamlined. Walk it off 30 minutes a day five times per week.

)55(Up the ante with these slimming secrets

Not too slow…

If you can sing while you walk, move it, you're not going fast enough.

Not too fast…

If you can't talk at all during your workout, you're going too fast.

Just right!

If you can mutter a few words—a conversation of single sentences is a good rule of thumb—but can't sing or gab like you would at the water-cooler, you've found the right momentum. Keep going.

)56(Keep up the good work

Research shows people often gain weight after 30 due to slacking off on their exercise and healthy eating habits, as well as sometimes due to a depressed mood. If you fear getting older means automatically inheriting your Aunt Gertrude's inner tube, stay on top of your workout efforts and healthy eating habits. Exercise will also go a long way to boost mood-improving serotonin levels in your brain to help you feel good and motivated to keep your sleek physique.

)57(Wear a pedometer

New research shows that pedometers create an awareness of your actual activity level and lead to increased physical activity.

)58(Don't get weighted down

Carrying hand weights or strapping on leg weights isn't a good idea. They can throw off your center of gravity and lead to injuries. Better: Swinging your arms as you walk can burn seventy extra calories an hour by making you work harder to swing your arms. To be sure you're in the swing, wear a couple of jingly bracelets and wave your fingertips so that your bracelets make a jingling sound as you walk.

)59(Tuck your tummy

Walk with good posture, tucking your butt under and sucking in your middle. Walking with good posture takes more energy and works your midsection muscles more than using a slouched, sloppy form. It also avoids neck and back pain!

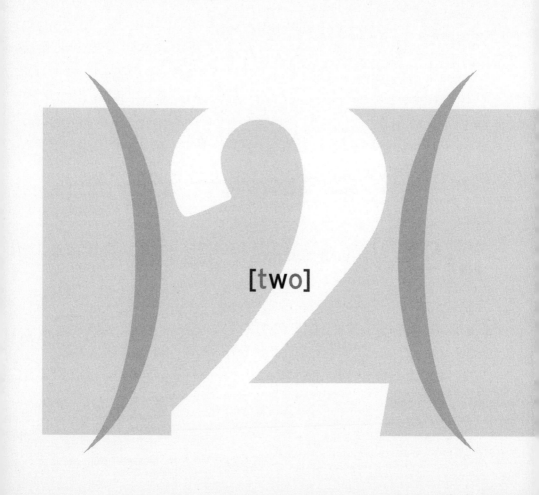

[two]

The Look Marvelous at the Office Plan

This is what the morning routine looks like for lots of us: Try on a pair of linen pants, take them off when the pleat doesn't lay properly. Try on a skirt, take it off when the zipper doesn't close. Curse. Don't eat breakfast, then grab a doughnut from the break room at the office at 10 A.M. because you're starving.

You can change this! These great shortcuts will help you feel calm, fit, and ready to take on anything. In this chapter, we'll tackle your belly, as well as the rest of your torso. Bra bulge—that dreaded roll of fat that seems to plant itself overnight (right after the baby has finally finished nursing or sometime after your 40th birthday) is just as bothersome as belly bulge. So fear not, your whole torso will benefit from the following tips. ~

Health and Beauty Bytes

)60(Sleep away calories

If you're losing winks, you may be gaining weight. The ideal time to snooze is 9 hours and 25 minutes, according to a national sleep organization. Not getting enough sleep alters the body's metabolic functions which can lead to weight gain and affect how the body processes food and stores carbohydrates. And when you're losing winks, you're more likely to down sugary foods and mega doses of carbohydrates to fight fatigued feelings. Here are some simple guidelines to lull you into dreamland.

) 61 (Add some zzz's

If you're not getting enough rest, adjust your schedule to go to bed earlier tonight and all week long. Next week, add another 15 to 30 minutes of rest to your schedule.

) 62 (Try the Early Bird Special

Eat dinner at least three hours before bedtime. Sleep expert Mark Rosekind, Ph.D., of Alertness Solutions in Cupertino, California, says your body needs time to digest before bed. Our busy schedules often mean pushing dinner until 8:30 P.M., or later, which makes it harder to fall asleep and get a restful night.

)63(Work out to fall asleep

Exercise one to two hours before bed. "Exercising close to bed disrupts sleep," Rosekind says. "It'll take you longer to fall asleep, and you'll experience lighter zzz's." But don't skip working out. Increased exercise improves sleep quality and is associated with falling asleep faster, especially for those who exercise in the morning.

)64(Create a technology-free zone

TVs, laptops, telephones, PDAs, and the like don't belong in the bedroom. Making your bedroom a sleep-only zone will help you sleep more soundly, according to the National Sleep Foundation.

) 65 (Set aside worry time

If your mind starts fretting the minute your head hits the pillow, set aside 15 minutes one hour before bed to write down whatever is bothering you in one column. In the other, write down the action you'll take tomorrow. Do this activity in another room besides the bedroom. Slip the list into a drawer to put it away for the day. If worries start creeping in once you hit the sack, use positive imagery to control worry. Thought blocking is another helpful aid. Every time you start thinking about what's bothering you, tell yourself "Stop! I will deal with this tomorrow." Try focusing your attention on the color black. Whenever your mind wanders, bring it back to a black screen. Before you know it, your worries will give way to zzz's.

)66(Avoid nighttime bathroom dashes

If you commonly wake up needing to pee, make sure you stop sipping three hours before bedtime so that your bedtime bathroom visit will be your last until the rooster crows. Also avoid diuretics such as alcohol or caffeine (that includes iced tea) and bladder irritants like spicy foods or citrus fruits—all will make you have to get up and go during the night.

Fitness Fun

)67(Take a break and crunch!

Think it's impossible to do an ab exercise if you work in a cubicle? Think again. Simply stand about two feet away from your desk with your feet about hip-width apart, shoulders relaxed, and pelvis in neutral. Bring your left knee up toward your right shoulder as you bring your bent arms down to meet it. Do this slowly and with focus about 10 times. Repeat on the other side. You should feel it right in your lower belly. This not only works your abs, but it gets your heart rate up a little, too!

)68(Get on the ball

Editors at one health and fitness magazine are rumored to not have desk chairs. They've swapped them for stability balls. Sitting on the ball encourages good posture (no slumped back and shoulders) and engages your abs, low back, legs, and glutes to help keep you stable. Plus, you'll burn more calories than if you sit in a regular office chair. Try this trick in front of the tube, too, to burn calories while watching your favorite sitcom.

)69(Pedal pushers

Lie on the floor, flat on your back. Keep your arms close to your torso. Tighten your midsection and lift your head, neck, and shoulders off the floor. Use your abs for stability. In this raised position, pull your left knee toward the chest and extend your right leg out straight several inches off the ground. Switch legs, making a pedaling motion as though you're riding a bike. Do two sets of 8 to 12 reps. One rep is complete when you've made a rotation with both feet.

)70(Try stomach smoothers

A physical therapist recommended doing this move while blow drying your hair and at every stoplight, to make your stomach look flatter. It can also be done while sitting at your desk—perhaps during those never-ending conference calls. Exhale and pull your belly button up and in while keeping your back straight. Hold for five seconds while continuing to breathe. Repeat 5 to 10 repetitions as often as you remember throughout the day to help tighten and tone your abdominal region.

Dos and Don'ts:

Here are some common mistakes that will get in the way of achieving your ultimate goal: a totally toned tummy.

)71(DON'T lace your fingers

Place both hands behind your head with fingertips just touching or slightly overlapped to support your head. Intertwining your fingers makes it easier to cheat and use your hands to lift your head up off the ground instead of your abs.

) 72 (DON'T be an overachiever

When it comes to toning your abs, you don't need to do 200 reps. In fact,
you shouldn't. Concentrate on achieving the correct number of reps and
doing the moves correctly. Slowing down is a better way to intensify
toning and achieve your goals than fatiguing your muscles with tons of
reps. Remember, form is more important than the rep number.

) 73 (DO contract your ab muscles

You gotta suck it in each and every time you do an ab move to do the
move correctly and to achieve slim and toned, rather than outward
bulging, abs. It's also smart to suck it up and in throughout the day to
engage the muscles for on-the-go toning.

) 74 (DON'T rush it

Ab work isn't the place to be a speed demon. It'll be over with soon
enough. Move slowly and stay in control so that momentum isn't powering
you through your ab workout. Most people tend to rush the moves at
the end of a set. Don't—this is exactly when you can reap the most benefit
from going slowly, steadily, and purposefully.

) 75 (DO let yourself down gently

The downward part of your ab exercise—when your leg, torso, or arm
moves down—is the easy part (kinda like jogging downhill). But this isn't
the time to rest. You get muscle work during this easy part of your workout,
so maximize it by moving slowly and gently, in a controlled manner.

)76(DON't forget to breathe

Oxygen fuels your muscles. If you clamp off your breathing during a move, your muscles will fatigue faster. Take deep belly breaths throughout your workouts, exhaling on the effort and inhaling on the easy section of the move.

)77(DON'T do the same exercises every time

Try new exercises offered in each section of this book to keep your muscles guessing. If you always do the same moves in the same order (for most of us, that's the basic crunch) your muscles will quickly adapt and the exercise will become less effective. To mix things up, reverse the order of your exercises, incorporate a new move, or do an extra rep or set. Just vary your workout slightly when any one move becomes too easy, to keep your workout from getting stagnant.

)78(Get moving on the weekends

Studies have shown that people actually move less on the weekends than they do during the week. Make a plan that involves going outside, taking a walk, or playing with your kids. Physical activity is much more relaxing than sitting on the couch. And if you are sitting on the couch, read a book or knit, rather than watching too much TV.

)79(Standing leg lifts

Stand with your back against a wall. Rest your palms against the wall and spread your feet several inches apart. Exhale and gently raise your right leg as high as you can. Hold. Inhale and slowly lower your leg. Lift forward 8 times. Then 8 to the side. Switch legs. Do two sets.

) 80 (Banish bra bulge

One of the first places the need to exercise shows is right below your underwire. Extra flesh squishing out below your bra band won't make your abs look trim. Take your exercise efforts up a notch, and, keep track of your calorie intake.

) 81 (Tone and uplift

Another common problem that can make your abs look less defined is breast sagging—an effect of gravity and time. While you cannot undo loose, sagging skin, you can work the pectoral muscles, which will help make breast skin look fuller and have a more lifted appearance. There will be more definition between your breasts and abs, making you look slimmer and more toned.

)82(Double crunches

Lie with your back on the floor, knees bent and heels in line with your buttocks. Place your hands behind your head for support, cradling it with your fingertips unlaced. Tighten your abs and make sure your lower back touches the floor. Gently lift your upper body, including your shoulder blades, off the mat, using your abs for strength. You should be reaching your torso toward your raised, bent knees. Lower back down to the mat. Do two sets of 8 to 15 reps.

)83(Leg pumps

Lie on your back with your knees bent and feet hip-width apart. Place your palms on your belly. Make sure your low back is flat against the floor, pelvis in neutral. Lift your right leg out straight and up (about as high as your bent knee) without arching your back, while simultaneously sucking in your gut. Slowly lower the leg back to the starting position. Do 8 to 15 reps on each side.

)84(Try ab-jabs

Lie on your back with your knees bent and feet flat on the floor. Tuck your arms in close to your chest and clench your fists under your chin— think boxer pose. Tighten your abs to gently lift your upper body so your shoulder blades are off the floor. Duck and weave like a boxer, making circles with your upper body. Keep your lower body stabilized and your arms up to prevent getting jabbed. Circle 8 to 10 times. Repeat in a counterclockwise direction.

)85(Don't eat sweets

Studies have shown that the most popular people in the office are the ones who keep candy on their desks. Sure, you love them, but does the candy love you? These treats have no nutritional value and once you indulge it's hard to keep from going back for more. Instead of derailing your stomach-slimming efforts, just say no to candy at work. Plus, hard candies cause you to swallow air leading to a bloated belly.

)86(Burn calories with protein

Eating protein for snacks and at every meal requires your body to burn more calories during digestion and absorption, helping you burn away belly fat and calories throughout the day.

)87(Snack on watery foods

Foods high in water content, such as asparagus and celery, are diuretics, which help flush out extra fluid from your body. Snack on these foods and you'll feel thinner and look leaner. Add a little protein (such as low-fat cheese or natural peanut butter) to help feel full. Another great low-cal snack: cottage cheese mixed with salsa. Skip the chips!

)88(Keep a big bottle on your desk

Not vodka. Not gin. Water. Your body needs 8 to 10 glasses of good old H_2O every day.

)89(Drink coffee

Research shows sipping coffee 30 minutes before a meal suppresses appetite by up to thirty-five percent and can even boost your metabolism. Just don't add lots of sugar! (But according to our low-carb gurus, feel free to pour in the cream!)

)90(Anticipate the post-lunch energy drag

The post-lunch energy dip is normal, but you may find yourself hitting the vending machine trying to get extra energy about that time. Instead, try isometric exercises, which will increase oxygen flow in the blood stream and help wake up your brain. Try pressing your knees against either side of your desk or pressing them together. Hold for 30 seconds and release. Repeat as needed.

)91(Don't skip breakfast

Studies show that people who skip breakfast are forty percent more likely to be overweight than those who eat something within one or two hours of waking up. Stick to something balanced in protein and complex carbs, such as eggs with whole-wheat toast or high-fiber cereal with milk.

)92(No soda!

Carbonated beverages (anything with little bubbles) are a source of air in the belly—and that extends your abdomen. Stick to water, a well-hydrated body is a thin body.

)93(Slow and steady

If you want to lose weight, you need to cut your caloric intake. To decrease the amount of calories you eat, shrink your portion size rather than foraging on "diet" foods (the cottage cheese, rice cracker, lettuce leaves route). Aim to eat 500 calories fewer per day to lose roughly one pound per week. Pay attention to serving sizes, which are listed on the backs of packaged foods and adjust your portions to more reasonable sizes. It's likely you'll find you're eating double the serving size of many foods.

)94(A little fiber goes a long way...

Fiber helps "clean out" the gastrointestinal tract. Eat fiber-rich foods such as dried fruits, prunes, prune juice, figs, fruits, and vegetables. Include plenty of fiber in your diet to stay regular, but also…

)95(Watch your fiber intake

…Be sure not to eat too much fiber in one sitting. Fiber can cause bloating because it expands once it's inside the digestive tract (think of how your shredded wheat expands in your cereal bowl). Limit your fiber intake to no more than about 10 grams at one sitting. Drink plenty of water (8 glasses per day) to help the fiber work properly.

)96(Plan healthy snacks

If you know you're likely to pig out while making dinner, make sure the only foods available are the raw veggies you're cutting up, some turkey, and a few whole wheat crackers. Take these healthy snacks with you to work and for the ride home too. These foods won't spike your insulin levels, which intensifies cravings. If you have healthy foods handy, you're unlikely to hit Krispy Kreme.

)97(Bring your own lunch

This not only saves you money, but also insures that you'll get a healthy meal. Your best bet? Turkey or cheese on whole-grain bread with tomato and lettuce, a salad or cup of soup, and a treat for dessert, such as two Hershey's Kisses or a piece of fruit.

workbook

Are your eyes bigger than your stomach?

Mom was right, most of us put far more on our plate (and then into our mouths) than we need. Eating out at restaurants with oversized bowls and plates and supersized portions can make you lose track of what's a reasonable portion size. Here are some sneaky ways to ensure you're getting a reasonable serving.

)98(Make your own plate

If you're lucky enough to have a guy who cooks, insist you serve yourself cafeteria style, scooping your own servings. Well-meaning men with spatulas may pile the plate the same for each of you. And after eating more, you will likely start heaping portions too high yourself.

)99(Weigh in

Start measuring your helpings with a food scale or measuring cups. Most people overestimate how much food they're eating by about one third. Once you get used to eye-balling the proper amount, you won't have to rely on the scale.

)100(Skip the guilt eating

If the "starving children" imagery guilts you into finishing a large plate of food, you are adding a lot of extra, unnecessary calories into your diet. Try reducing your portion, or set a mental limit on how much you will consume.

) 101 (Put pasta in a cereal bowl

Pasta bowls are notoriously huge. Put your dinner serving in a cereal bowl—you'll actually get the proper amount of noodles and it will fill your dish more than if you used a large one. Want to add something else to your repast? Transfer the noodles back to the pasta bowl and add a protein as well as vegetables for the healthiest and most filling meal of all.

) 102 (Let your fist be your guide

It's a good rule of thumb that your meal (if you're adhering to the six meal a day plan) should be roughly the size of two fists—a snack should be the size of one fist.

)103(Don't eat like your kids

Your kids may prefer a steady diet of high sugar, high fat foods, but they're a lot less likely to gain weight if they learn to eat like you, rather than vice versa. In other words, don't let them (or yourself) eat lots of processed snack foods like goldfish crackers, chips, or soda. Get them in the habit of eating well. Focus on eating three meals a day that include a protein and lots of complex carbs (veggies and whole grains). Snacks can be fruit and a protein. They'll grow up healthy and so will you.

)104(Top it off

The best way to round out a fast food meal is with skim milk (even if it's chocolate flavored!) or yogurt (make sure it doesn't have too much sugar) and lots of water to help get rid of all the salt those meals typically contain.

)105(Choose texture, color, and flavor

If you're even slightly overweight, chances are you're used to highly flavorful foods and a lot of them. If you're trying to lose weight, you need to reduce your portion size to a more reasonable amount and therefore you'll get less flavor in your effort to reduce calories. Don't fall into the diet trap and start eating flavorless "diet" foods, advises Susan Schiffman, Ph.D., a flavor expert and scientific director for the Sense of Smell Foundation in New York City. Eating like an anemic rabbit is only going to ensure that you don't stick with your weight loss efforts. Instead, use your sense of smell to your advantage to make your weight control efforts a success. Flavor your food with citrus, garlic, onion, and other flavors and spices to help satisfy your taste buds.

)106(**Avoid clingy fabrics**

If your bra roll is noticeable through your tops, avoid tight-fitting, body-hugging fabrics. Looser cotton fabric won't accentuate your worry zone.

)107(**Forget the demi**

Buying new bras? Try non-demi cup styles which offer a fuller cup and more coverage for a sleeker line under your shirts. Bras without seams and cotton bras without lace look the best under tailored tops.

)108(Skip stripes

Horizontal stripes add bulk. A TV celebrity dresser once told me that when dressing a busty broadcaster, she wouldn't dream of using stripes. But she's a big fan of solid colors and wearing a jacket to help slim the breast area. Wearing a V-neck (not a cleavage-showing, low-dipping one) can also help create a vertical line, which is slimming.

)109(Wear a jacket

Long jackets that hit below the hips help you look longer and leaner and bring the eye away from your abs. Stay away from jackets with wide shoulders, as that will give you a "big" look. Instead, try pinstripes or stitching that brings attention to the design of the cloth, rather than the jacket's cut.

)110(Go for double breasted

Double-breasted styles minimize bust. This will make you look slimmer all over and the double rows of buttons create the illusion of a waist.

)111(Get steamed

Iron your clothes. Wrinkled clothing doesn't lay flat or drape the body. The creases make it appear that the garment is puckering and pulling because it doesn't fit right, when in fact all it needs is pressing.

workbook

)112(Slim styling

If you're trying to hide what you'll soon tone up, save these styles until you've whittled your middle:

The no, no	Reason
Boy cut pants	Emphasize a wide waist
Hiphuggers	Draw attention to the belly
Capris	Create an unbalanced look
Boxy cuts	Make the body look wider
Horizontal stripes	Emphasize width
Bolero cropped jackets	Make you look wider
Heavy knits	Bulk you up

Did you know?

) 113 (Stress packs on pounds

As if your everyday, jam-packed, crazy-making schedule isn't enough to worry about, belly chub may be a sign of stress. In one Yale University study, otherwise slender women with excess weight around their midline were shown to not cope with stress well. They had more of the stress hormone cortisol pumping through their veins, and were quicker to anger than other women. Another study found greater exposure to cortisol among men and women with extra flesh around the middle may have played a role in contributing to their greater abdominal fat deposits. Belly fat has been shown to increase the risk of health problems like diabetes, heart disease, stroke, and cancer. And it doesn't look too good hanging over your string bikini underwear either.

) 114 (Laughter library

To cope, zap frazzled feelings before stress overload causes you to store visceral fat below the abdominal muscles. Keep a collection of your favorite jokes, cartoons, comedians, or hilarious sitcoms and movies to lighten up a taxing day. Laughter, after all, is the best medicine.

) 115 (Take a hobby holiday

Carve out time for a hobby to have some fun and help dissolve stress that could be contributing to the fat stored around your torso.

) 116 (Use your resources

If stress is a real issue for you, it's a good idea for your health and your looks to seek out professional counseling or a stress-management workshop. Your workplace may offer a stress-management class or your health insurance could cover the cost of psychotherapy to help you take control of stress.

) 117 (Take a short vacation

When you just can't deal, give stress the slip. Whether you're distraught over the spat with your best friend, the numbers on the scale, or getting passed over for a promotion—sometimes it can all just be too stressful to deal with. Press the escape key. Putting your problems on hold by taking a mental vacation can rekindle your spirit and recharge your emotional batteries. While it's hard to book a one-way ticket to paradise in seconds, you can reap the benefits of an island oasis in just 15 minutes. Try visualization to tap into the same relaxation response that a real vacation gives, without spending a dime. Here's how:

First, find a quiet, private place and sink into a chair with both feet on the ground. Or, lie down. Now close your eyes and picture yourself walking barefoot in the sand with the surf lapping at your heels. Feel the warm sunshine on your face and hear the ocean waves crashing against the beach. Stop to build a sand castle or gather seashells and gaze out on the endless sea of blue as you breathe deeply and take in the warm, salty mist of the ocean air. Visit this or your very own special place in your mind's eye whenever you need an instant way to say so-long to stress.

) 118 (Practice gratitude

Whenever life seems like too much, spend a few minutes thinking of all the things in life you have to be thankful for. In fact, start every day with this attitude of gratitude to put it all in perspective!

) 119 (Get sized for a new bra

An estimated seven in ten women wear the wrong size bra. That excess flesh squishing out from your underwire may be easily solved by having a fitter measure you and suggest the right-sized bra. In fact, a properly-fitted bra can make your torso look leaner. Go to a department store, lingerie shop, or even an outlet that sells underwear and ask to be fitted. It'll only take a few minutes for the pro to slip the tape around you and size you up correctly.

The Yoga Workout

Yoga works your whole body—mind, body, and spirit. These poses will engage your abs as well as help you feel relaxed and renewed. Stretches that elongate your abdominals will help create that strong, lean middle. Doing yoga regularly will improve your flexibility, posture, and strength, while giving you that fringe benefit you're looking for—sculpted ab muscles. Try these yoga moves.

)120(Mountain tilt

Stand with your arms at your side and your feet hip-width apart. Your toes should face forward. Raise your arms above your head, pointing your fingers upwards. Bend sideways at the waist, extending up and out to your left. Hold for a few seconds and return to center. Repeat on the right side. Do 3 to 5 times.

)121(Triangle pose

Stand tall with your feet 3-feet apart. Turn your left foot out 90 degrees while keeping your right foot pointing forward. Extend your arms out to either side at shoulder height. Bend to your right at your waist, keeping your chest facing forward, and place your right hand on your shin as your left arm reaches up. Your eyes should look skyward (if this hurts your neck, look down). Hold for 15 seconds and return to the starting position. Switch feet and sides. Do 3 times on each side.

)122(Torso stretch

Lie on your belly, hands flat on the floor close to your chest. Point your toes. Lift your upper body by pressing the tops of your feet and shins into the floor as you press your hands into the floor and straighten your arms. Breathe. Hold for 40 seconds.

)123(Bending forward pose

Sit with your legs together stretched straight in front of you. Point your toes. Inhale and stretch toward your toes with your finger tips, keeping your body long and extended. Hold for thirty seconds. Breathe normally. Return to the starting position. Repeat.

)124(Butterfly pose

Sit on the floor stretching straight up through your spine. Bring the heels of your feet together, with your knees bent and pointing out to the sides. Let your legs open towards the floor to a position where you are comfortable. Hold your feet in your hands and slowly stretch forward. Lower your head toward your toes as far as you can. Hold for 5 seconds then return to the starting position. Repeat 3 times to help open hips and warm up.

)125(Bridge pose

Lie on your back with your knees bent and feet hip-width apart. Rest your arms at your side. Using your abdominals, lift your hips as far as you can off the floor. Your head, shoulders, and arms should remain on the floor. Keep your thighs parallel. Hold. Repeat 5 times.

)126(Locust pose

Lie on your stomach so that your chin is on the floor and your arms are extended in front of you. Engage your abs. Inhale and lift your arms, chest, head, legs, and feet off the floor. Hold for 3 seconds then slowly lower to the floor. Repeat 5 times.

)127(Cat pose

Get on all fours and look straight ahead with your back as flat as a table. Exhale and arch your back upwards while tucking your chin to your chest. Inhale and arch your back downwards, swaying the low back as you look toward the ceiling. Repeat up to 5 times.

)128(Yoga crunches

Lie on your back and bring your knees to your chest. Rest your hands over your head on the floor behind you and raise your legs with feet flexed toward the ceiling. Use your ab muscles to slowly guide your legs downward. Stop when you feel your back arching. Hug your legs to your chest again. Repeat. Build up to 10 in a row.

workbook

Dos and Don'ts

)129(DO go slow

Using slow, controlled motions will ensure momentum isn't at work, but that your ab muscles are. Zooming through the moves won't ensure as much muscle recruitment or involvement. If an exercise seems too easy, check your form and try again s-l-o-w-l-y. Chances are a minor correction to your form and a slower pace will make a big difference in how effective the exercise is.

)130(DON'T hold your breath

Your breath is essential in yoga and during exercise in general. Taking deep inhalations and exhalations will not only wake up the muscles but also help you stretch deeper when performing yoga. And your breath with also help stabilize and strengthen you for other core-building moves. Whenever you feel like you've stretched as far as you can or cannot do one more rep, take a deep inhale. Feel your muscles sink into a deeper stretch or help you push through one more rep.

)131(DO say "Om"

In yoga, the mind-body connection is essential. Take a few moments to clear your mind and get in touch with your body before starting yoga moves. Take deep, cleansing breaths, and listen to your body. Only do a little more than you thought you could and tackle more next time. At the end of your work-out, use your cool down to close your eyes and connect within for a more peaceful, centered you.

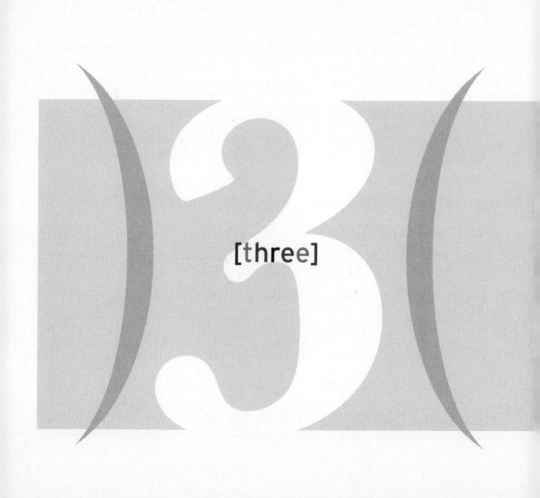

[three]

The Fabulous Party Plan

The following tips will work for any soiree—a high school reunion, an office holiday party, or your favorite niece's Bat Mitzvah. You deserve to look and feel your best at any special event. And hey, if you're paying big money for a great outfit, you'll want to bring your spectacular abs along to the party. ~

)132(Stop fat talk

"Do I look fat?" does nothing to make others think your abs are buff, nor does it help your self confidence. Turn off the negative tape in your head and tune into a more positive self-perception. If your girlfriends start in, change the subject fast so you all don't end up wallowing in a junk food self-pity party that will dash your efforts at getting a sexier stomach—not to mention maintaining your self-esteem.

)133(Sweep your hair into a ponytail

What does your hairdo have to do with sexier abs? Plenty. The way you style your hair can make you look longer and leaner. Try an updated ponytail: Gently tease the crown using a comb, smooth your hair straight back with your hands (without a part), and secure a high ponytail at the middle of your head. Gently loosen the hair at the crown for a fuller look. Try teasing the tail below the elastic band for a perky ponytail. Or the curl the ends under with a single hot roller. Be sure to gently finger and separate the ponytail once it's curled for a more natural look.

)134(Take an anti-gas tablet

Over-the-counter anti-gas medication containing simethicone helps relieve some stomach swelling caused by taking in too much air or eating belly-bloating foods. Follow package directions.

)135(Visualize your beautiful bod

Before you head to the refrigerator or eat another office party doughnut, close your eyes, let go of your breath, and imagine yourself choosing instead to have either a healthy snack or just a glass of water. If you're really hungry, visualize a healthy meal, such as soup or a salad and some fish. Keep breathing deeply and further visualize getting into exactly the kind of dress (or size jeans) that you would wear if you were at the weight you desire. Visualization has been shown to help people reach their goals.

)136(There you glow

Shimmery body creams called highlighters help you to sparkle. Tiny light-reflecting particles give a subtle summery shine to make your totally-toned abs stand out. Liquid body lotion and cream forms work best for easy smoothing and effortless blending. Try accentuating your obliques by applying an extra coat with upward strokes to the exterior edge of the muscles when wearing body-bearing clothes. Hues range from soft, pearly shades for fair skin tones to deeper, coppery colors that make olive skin tones really shine. Pale, powdery pinks are best for ruddy skin tones.

)137(Suck it in

Throughout the party, remember to engage your ab muscles. Think of pulling your belly button up and in as if you're zipping a pair of tight jeans. This will help you flatten your abs, maintain balance and control, and instantly get a longer, leaner, and more uplifted appearance.

)138(Help minimize stomach swell by getting more calcium

Help minimize stomach swell by getting more calcium A study in the American Journal of Obstetrics and Gynecology showed a daily dose of 1,200 mg of calcium decreased premenstrual syndrome (PMS) discomforts. By warding off the emotional tension and mood swings, you will probably not end up with your spoon in a pint of Ben and Jerry's Chunky Monkey, which will go a long way toward your goal to whittle your middle.

)139(Take a salt soak

Shake sea salt or Epsom salts into your bath water. Salt water reverses osmosis, drawing out water retention. While eating salt makes you retain water, soaking in the potassium, magnesium, and bromide in salt soaks helps draw out water retention, detoxifying the cells and banishing bloating.

)140(Look five pounds thinner by changing your hairstyle

Wide hair can make you look wide all over. Ask for a style with pieces that are cut into your face. Use your blow drier to give a little height to the top of your hair, which makes you look longer and leaner. Stylists also recommend face-framing layers and long, fine bangs for a slimming effect. Steer clear of thick bangs that add bulk.

)141(Try this red carpet celebrity secret

A personal trainer to the stars once told me celebrities slather Preparation-H on their stomachs before slipping into a body-baring dress for the Oscars. As unappealing as it sounds, the topical cream shrinks swollen skin tissues, temporarily making the abs look sleeker and sexier. And I believe it might do some good for an extended pouch because dermatologists have recommended the same thing for an in-a-pinch fix for puffy areas under the eyes.

)142(While you're blow-drying...

You can sneak ab exercises into your beauty routine. If you bend over to blow the underside of your hair, make sure you contract your abs and tuck your pelvis under while you're in the forward bend (keep your shoulders relaxed and back flat, too). This will help your posture when you stand up. Standing and reaching up with the blow dryer and a brush? Once again, make sure your pelvis is tucked and your abs contracted to be sure you're standing properly and in neutral.

)143(Hang over your bed

Heading out to a fabulous fiesta? Before you dress, lie on your bed with your upper back, shoulders, neck, and head all hanging over the side. Keep your pelvis tucked in neutral as you let gravity lengthen your spine. Hold this for a few minutes. You won't add any inches (officially), but the great stretch will certainly give you a long and leaner look for the evening's event.

) 144 (Sing

Loud, energetic singing works your diaphragm, a muscle in your torso that only works properly if you stand properly and exercise it regularly. So let loose like a diva in the shower or the car, it will help you to naturally stand taller. (You could also practice yodeling, but I'll assume you'd rather imitate Madonna than Hans the Sheepherder)

Fitness Fun

) 145 (Don't sit down!

On the phone? Keep walking, baby, even if it's just to pace your living room. Studies show that taking 10,000 to 15,000 steps every day is a step (get it?) toward maintaining your proper weight. So, keep moving whenever possible—it will go a long way to helping the fat melt off your belly.

) **146** (Belly ball

Lie on your back, knees bent and feet flat on the floor. Hold a small basketball, volleyball, or medicine ball (no more than three to five pounds) to your chest, keeping your elbows bent and close to your sides. Tighten your abs, pulling your belly button in and up, and lift your upper body so your shoulder blades are off the floor. In this position, toss the ball up in the air. Catch it, then slowly lie back down—moving one vertebra at a time. Repeat. Do one set of 8 to 15 reps.

)147(Showgirl kicks

Sit with your feet flat on the floor, knees bent and legs together. Lean back so that your toes just touch the floor, supporting your weight with your elbows behind you and palms flat on the floor. Drop your legs to the right, then left. Kick your lower legs upwards as high as you can. Draw your knees back in and drop your legs to the left, then right and back to the left, then kick up again. Do 8 to 15 times.

workbook

)148(Improve your posture

Want to look instantly longer, leaner, and more toned—ten pounds thinner even? Of course you do, so mind your posture. Anytime you straighten yourself upwards, you're working the postural muscles at your core and that means you're fighting against that slouchy look—rolled shoulders, bowed back, saggy stomach. Standing tall won't just make your mother happy, good posture is good for your ab muscles, back health, and breathing. You use your abdominal muscles and back muscles to stand up straight. If your abs are weak, it will make your back work harder to compensate. And that can lead to back injury or pain. Practicing good posture helps promote strong abs and back. In turn, strong abdominal muscles help support your torso, keeping your spine in proper alignment. When it comes to perfect posture, there are several simple adjustments to make. Your mother probably tried to drill most of them into your head as a child. Mine had a neighbor who was a physical therapist "drop by" to give us a proper posture pep talk. It served me well (despite a lot of eye rolling), so I'll pass it on to you. Try practicing every time you brush your teeth and as you remember throughout the day. Soon standing (and sitting) tall will be second nature:

· **Firmly plant your feet on the ground**, finding a comfortable balance point with your weight evenly distributed between the pads of your feet and your toes.

· **Take a deep breath** and lift up through the top of your head, straightening your back. Feel pressure release from your low back.

- **Look straight ahead.** Your chin should be in line with the floor or pointing slightly downward. Feel your jaw and neck muscles relax.

- **Relax your shoulders** and gently roll them backwards, opening up the chest area. Feel stronger and take deeper, clearer breaths.

- **Contract your abs**, pull in your belly button, and slightly rotate your hip bones backwards so that your buttocks tuck under you. Feel your abs and butt getting firmer every time you practice.

- **Straighten you spine** as though you're a marionette on a string and feel the relief you find from taking pressure off your back.

)149(Uneven push ups

Place a phone book on the floor. Now put a dumbbell in your right hand and place it on top of the phone book. Put your left hand on the floor and assume a plank (or push-up) position: feet together, arms straight, hands under your shoulders. Slowly lower yourself toward the ground with your back straight. Return to start, pushing yourself back up into a plank. Do a modified push up with your knees on the ground if this is too difficult. Do one set of 10 reps. Repeat on the opposite side.

)150(Be the Alps

The Mountain pose helps you center and adjust your alignment. Stand with your arms at your side, feet together or slightly apart, and head looking forward. Keep your legs straight without locking your knees. Relax your shoulders and arms, keeping them straight next to your sides. Your shoulders should be relaxed and slightly back, not slumped forward. Gently shift your weight and move your body slightly forward until you find a tall, comfortable position where you feel centered, balanced, and relaxed, but strong. You should feel as though someone is pulling a string attached to the top of your head, lifting you into a proper stance. Your weight should be evenly distributed between the heels, toes, and balls of your feet. Stay in the pose for several minutes, feeling your breath move in and out.

)151(Sideways crunches

Lie on your right side. Bend both knees and extend your right arm, resting your head on the outstretched arm. For stability, be sure the hourglass curve of your waistline is pressed into the mat. Crunch up, contracting the muscles on your right side. Lift your upper body toward your raised hip. Do 8 to 15 crunches on each side.

)152(Incline fly/Pullover combination

Lie with two large pillow shams under your upper back. Hold a
five-pound dumbbell in each hand and extend both arms straight up
over the middle of your chest. Start lowering your arms out to the
sides (palms facing one another) to form a T. Raise them back to the
starting position. Go immediately into a pullover: lower the weights over
your head with your arms slightly bent and palms facing one another.
Keep your back flat—be sure it doesn't arch. Return to start. Do two
sets of 10.

) 153 (Side-to-side crisscrosses

Lie on the floor in the traditional crunch position with your arms
behind your head, fingers touching and your feet flat on the floor,
shoulder-width apart. Extend your left leg up with your toe pointed
toward the ceiling. Bend your right leg in toward your torso. Lift
your head off the floor, still supporting your neck with your fingertips.
Touch your right elbow to your left knee. Return to center. Extend
your right leg as high as you can with toe pointed. Now lift and touch
your left elbow to your right knee. Do 8 to 15 times per side.

) 154 (Take twist time

Do side twists while brushing your teeth, talking on the phone, waiting
in line—all those lost minutes add up to big opportunities to slim your
sides. Side twists help engage the obliques and target the common
trouble spot: side bulge.

)155(Toe taps

Lie on your back, hands at your sides and feet on the floor. Tighten
your abs and point your toes. Now lift your legs up and then tap your
toes down on the floor. Do three sets of 8 to 15 reps. Gradually work
your taps father away from the body for more of a challenge.

)156(Side twists

Lie on your back and extend your arms out fully on either side.
Bend your knees to a ninety-degree angle and elevate them slightly.
Simultaneously drop your knees to the right (keeping the leg position
open and extended) and turn your head to the left. Hold for 30
seconds. Return knees and head to the center and twist in the
opposite direction. Do two sets of 12 twists.

)157(Raised crunches

Lie on your right side with your knees bent and your right elbow in line with your right shoulder. Put your left hand behind your head. Tighten your abs and raise your entire body so that your weight is supported by your right forearm and the right lower leg and knee. Point your left leg and extend it at hip height. Maintain the position while bending your left knee up so it's in line with your hips and crunch your left elbow to the left knee. Straighten your leg, keeping it at hip height. Do two sets of 10 to 15 reps on each side.

)158(Try a Bosu

Half a fitness ball glued onto a solid platform, the Bosu is a hot new exercise tool that forces you to stabilize your deepest abdominal muscles while you do all sorts of exercise, including yoga, aerobics, Pilates, and strength training. Each Bosu comes with an instructional video and you will not believe how hard you'll have to use your abs just to stand still on this deceptive new contraption.

Nutrition Nuggets

)159(Use the eighty percent rule

In many Asian cultures, people learn to stop eating when they feel eighty percent full rather than one-hundred percent stuffed. This is a sense perception and not an actual measurement. To follow the rule, you need to eat slowly and be aware of when you almost feel full. Don't worry! You won't feel hungry, instead, you'll feel satisfied. If you're hungry a couple of hours later, once again, have a snack that also satisfies you eighty percent. In this way, you'll eat less over the course of the day and will never over-stuff your stomach.

)160(Prevent overeating tonight

Don't starve yourself while getting ready. Eating a small and healthy meal ensures that you won't overindulge when you finally get to the table tonight, packing yourself full of excess calories and fat.

)161(Beware of surprising belly bloaters

Any day you plan to show off your toned abs, avoid gassy foods that will bloat your belly. Eating beans, garlic, and some legumes can cause excess gas. Some gas is normal—some doctors say releasing gas from seven to eleven times per day is typical, even though it's generally not invited.

)162(Take the small plate

Use appetizer plates instead of dinner plates to make yourself feel like you're filling the plate, even though you'll be eating less food than you would with a large dish.

)163(Think flavor when cooking

Treat yourself to flavored rubs and spices. Grow fresh herbs on your windowsill so mouth-watering flavors are always just a snip away. Some culinary favorites include flat leaf parsley, rosemary, basil, dill, chives, cilantro, and oregano. Adding more flavor to your food will help you eat less because you'll enjoy smaller more savory servings.

)164(Sip on the rocks

Add ice to your daily eight glasses of water per day. The body works harder to get cold water up to body temperature so that it can be absorbed through the stomach lining. You can expect to burn an extra sixty calories thanks to the cubes.

)165(Choose a tall glass rather than a short one

There is an illusion at work. When people drink from squat tumblers, they often think they're enjoying less than they are—which can lead to consuming more calories and possibly more alcohol than you mean to. Try pouring ¾ cup of water into a short glass to see how much one serving is. It's probably less than you think.

) 166 (Know what you eat—and how much

Keep a food diary to accurately record what you eat day-to-day. That means counting what you'd rather not admit to: the two handfuls of chocolate chips that you snitched from the pantry in a weak moment and that half-cup of ice cream you ate with those strawberries.

) 167 (Nuts and water

Before you head out the door, have a handful of almonds or cashews and two glasses of water. This will help you handle the first drink of the evening and stave off noshing on the first thing you see at the party.

) 168 (Is it buffet?

Choose one thing you really want to try (okay, maybe two) then cover your plate with veggies and lean sources of protein such as meat, fish, and hard cheese (but just a few cubes).

) 169 (Split your drinks with water

A good rule to avoid empty calories as well as over-drinking? Have one glass of wine or spirits and then follow it with a glass of water. Repeat. You'll have your two glasses to enjoy, but the water will help you pace yourself and fill your tummy.

)170(Three bites

Want to splurge on a fabulous piece of cake? Order a slice to split with a friend, then plan to eat three bites. The first one is for taste, the second is to satisfy you, and the third one is to finish. All done and you haven't overeaten!

) 171 (Watch your sodium

Anyway you shake it, salt intake causes you to retain fluids. Mega doses of snack foods (pretzels, chips, salty crackers) can cause you to look and feel puffy and swollen all over.

) 172 (Sip cranberry juice

If you notice you can't get your rings off the morning after you dined out, and your watch, bracelets, or shoes are fitting tighter, salt is likely to blame for causing you to retain fluid and contributing to your overall balloon-like feeling. Help flush the salt out of your system by drinking plenty of water mixed with cranberry juice, a diuretic.

workbook

Healthy ways to stop overeating

A recent Tufts University study found half of the average population's annual weight gain occurs during the last six weeks of the year. It's also well understood that most people overeat when faced with supersized restaurant portions, which means when you're dining out, your belly will feel and look bloated. To keep your cravings under control at a holiday party or when eating out:

)173(Stick with fork foods

Foods that require a fork to eat are less fattening than ones you can pick up and nibble (i.e. bacon-wrapped scallops vs. grilled scallops, fries vs. mashed potatoes, chicken fingers vs. marinated grilled chicken). Eliminate finger foods for a fast way to trim the fat.

)174(Wear your little black dress

Slip into something tight and sexy. You'll think twice about overstuffing yourself at the buffet table.

)175(Not too close

Choose to stand and chat away from the appetizers. Keeping a healthy distance will ensure you don't have your hand in the chip bowl all night long.

)176(Kudos to the hostess

When your grandmother tries pushing another helping onto your plate, tell her it was so delicious you couldn't possibly eat another morsel. Admit to dieting, and she'll just pile it on.

)177(Know what you love and stick to it

Everyone has their favorite treat, so if yours is candy, don't bother with ice cream, cake, or chips. Choose the one treat that you know will satisfy you and plan to have small amounts of it a few times a week at a time when you can really enjoy it (not when you're sitting at your desk or driving in your car).

)178(Stock up on veggies

Make sure vegetables and fruits occupy more room on your plate than meat or grains. On days when you want your abs to look their best, be sure to minimize refined carbs, high-fat dairy, and sweets. Focusing on lean protein foods helps your abdominal muscles really show through.

) 179 (Wear a great belt

Lots of waist-conscious women shy away from belts, thinking that they will bring attention to the problem area. But, oh no, *ma chérie*, belts actually give the illusion of a waist by cutting the body in half and creating a curve where one may not exist. You can always opt for the one-line-fools-all rule by wearing black from head to toe, but if you want to create the illusion of an hourglass figure (and, after all, that is what most men want), wear a belt to create a waist.

)180(Go long!

Try longer, tank-style tops with built-in bras instead of skimpier and shorter styles that hit right in the bra bulge zone. This will help cover more of your trouble zone for a slimmer, sleeker appearance.

)181(Try long boots

Tall boots with a thin heel create a long look, especially under skirts. Stay away from skirts with pleats, which never sit well on a belly unless it's extraordinarily long and lean.

) 182 (Go monochromatic

Choose monochromatic or monotone clothing to elongate the body, creating a long, lean line. Classic colors like camel, brown, black, gray, and navy work best. Add color with accessories: a purse, boots, shoes, or scarf.

) 183 (Gravitate toward wide legs

Wide-legged jeans and pants help conceal bulges in the tummy, hips, and thighs, making your whole midsection look sleeker and sexier. Width at the ankle balances the midsection, whereas skinny, pencil pants make the midsection appear wider.

)184(Buy a larger size

I know, the smaller the number on your clothing tag, the better your psychological state. But buying up one size can make you look 10 pounds lighter. Talk about a psychological advantage. Cut the tags out when you get home to avoid post-traumatic stress disorder every time you see the bigger number.

)185(Seek Chevron stripes

Chevron stripes that are directed like a "V" visually create a slimmer mid-section.

workbook

)186(Did you know?

Personal shoppers are available at major department stores. If your goal is to dress thinner, schedule time with a professional shopper to help you make better choices in the dressing room. Simply call a week in advance and ask to speak with a personal shopper. The objectivity of the shopper will aid you in finding styles that best flatter your shape. The shopper can also be budget-conscious, helping you to select clothing styles and colors that will have staying power in your wardrobe and won't go out of style 5 minutes after you buy them.

)187(Try wrap-around styles

A TV wardrobe stylist once told me wrap-around skirts, shirts, tops, and dresses are slimming because they create a diagonal line. The sarong effect a wraparound skirt lends to the waistline helps hide the tummy.

)188(Get a shaper

Try an up-to-date shaper (no, not a girdle). Boy-cut briefs with a slimming front panel help hold in the tummy. It'll remind you to suck it in and help you carry yourself better. A bonus: it's a great reminder not to overstuff yourself with appetizers.

)189(Did you know?

Breast support is essential for keeping your breasts from down shifting.
A regular bra does not give adequate breast support during high impact
exercise (aerobics, jogging, jumping rope). Find a comfortable sports bra
that minimizes bounce to wear during exercise. Some bras are rated for
varying levels of support so you can choose the right one for your sport.

workbook

Dos and Don'ts

)190(DON'T choose chunky-heeled, boxy-toed shoes

Thin heels are better, such as pointed-toe and thinly heeled boots paired with jeans or pants.

)191(DON'T select boxy cut jackets

This style will give your upper body a bulky look.

)192(DON'T bare just because you dare

Try tummy-flattening swimsuits designed to minimize the tummy for a trimmer look overall. These are made by Land's End and other quality swimwear manufacturers.

)193(DO try monochromatic dressing

This will visually lengthen and slim your figure, creating a long, lean line.

Add a splash of color in accessories—shoes, handbag, necklace or bracelet.

)194(DO wear a thong

Thongs prevent bunchy panty lines that make you look bulky.

)195(DO, for all our sakes, skip the painted-on pants

Outlining every curve means every bulge gets underscored too.

)196(DON'T wear ankle-strapped shoes

They make your ankles look thicker and you look weighed down.

)197(DO choose low-cut underwear

Practice bending over in the mirror to make sure your underwear doesn't ride up and peek out of the waistband of your low-rise jeans.

)198(DON'T wear low-slung pants

Wait until you've said so-long to those love-handles. Even if you tuck in your shirt, side bulges still show and look larger than in regular pants.

)199(DO try tankinis

This style lets you flash a peek at your abs without revealing your entire stomach.

) 200 (Give flowing fabrics the pass

Skip romantic, gossamer fabrics and go for heavier weights that smooth over the body without puckering.

Fabulous Party Exercise Plans— 10-Minute Cardio Workouts

Before a cardio workout, always be sure to warm up your muscles before you really get moving. Try walking up and down a couple flights of stairs, jogging in place, twisting your torso, stretching your calves. While experts are divided on whether warming up prevents injuries, a quick warm up certainly is an effective alarm clock for "cold" muscles—helping you get fired up and ready to move.

Oh, and about those calorie counts. If you're sitting and watching TV, you'll burn slightly less than one calorie per minute (that's less than sixty calories per hour). Stand up and start doing something, such as cleaning the house or exercising, and you'll burn on average about five times that number!

But there's even better news: The body is a machine that follows the laws of physics—the more you sit, the less you burn; the more you move, the more you burn. Your body keeps burning extra calories after you exercise, which is why even 10-minute workouts can make a big difference to your figure.

)201(Jump rope

No time? Supercharge your workout, getting an intense, speedy workout. Olympic athletes and celebrity personal trainers swear by this. Do it up to four times a week. It'll help you burn calories and tone all-over—core, arm, legs, etc. If you've got two left feet, try using a pretend jump rope to prevent tangling your workout with mis-steps. Wear cross-trainers and warm up beforehand. Start jumping for one minute and work up to ten for a real cardio kick. You'll wonder how you ever jumped rope all through recess! For variety, try hopping on one leg, then the other. Try doing a double jump before the rope comes full circle. Then resume standard skipping..

) 202 (Jumping jacks

Similar to jumping rope, jumping jacks work the whole body and give you a cardio blast in a short time frame. Plus they help create a long, lean look. Start by doing jumping jacks for 1 minute and work up to 10 minutes. For variety, try twisting your upper body to the left during one jumping jack, back to center, and then to the right on the next jump to get some targeted side-slimming action.

) 203 (Walk your dog (or someone else's)

No, we don't mean take him two houses down and turn around. Take him on a jog and he'll help you keep a fast pace on hills and be a good motivator to keep with it everyday, twice a day. He'll bug you when it's walk time, and there's no telling him "not today"—your exercise excuses won't work on a pooch.

) 204 (Do a series of lunges, squats, and push-ups

Want to get a full-body strength workout in just 10 minutes? Do three sets of lunges (Step forward with your right leg and bend your knees, step back, and repeat on the other side. Do 20 reps.), squats (Stand with your feet hip-distance apart, bend your knees and hips and come into a sitting position, hold for one second, then come up. Repeat 20 times.), and push-ups (Begin with your hands on the floor, just beneath your shoulders, and knees—or toes, if you can—on the ground. Bend your elbows and bring your chest to the floor. Push up and repeat 5-10 times.)

) 205 (Sun salutes

Do five yoga sun salutations—moves that are done in a series to stretch and strengthen every muscle of the body, including the heart. They are: Mountain pose, arch back (inhale), forward bend (exhale), extended forward bend (inhale), forward bend (exhale), lunge back and arch (inhale), downward facing dog (exhale), cobra (inhale), plank pose (exhale), lunge and arch (inhale), forward bend (exhale), extended forward bend (inhale), forward bend (exhale), come up, extend and arch back (inhale), return to mountain (exhale).

) 206 (Dance!

Turn on the radio or your CD player and pump up the volume and your heart rate for at least four songs (Okay, so that's probably more like 12 minutes). This is exactly what 80s music was made for.

) 207 (Stairs, stairs, stairs!

Perhaps the best piece of exercise equipment of all time is a flight of stairs. Think it only works your butt and legs? Think again. Maintaining your balance as you run (quickly!) up a flight of stairs will burn calories and keep your abs toned because, in order to stay balanced as you move, your abs need to be engaged. So, find a flight of stairs and have at 'em!

)208(Kickbox

Even if you're no Ali, you can put together a boxing routine that will get your blood pumping. Combine and alternate the following moves for 10 minutes:

- **Boxers' shuffle**—bounce from side to side, making sure your feet are always moving
- **Jabs**—punch straight out from your body
- **Crosses**—punch across your body
- **Hooks**—take your arm out to the side and then bring it around past your face
- **Uppercuts**—bring your arm down in front of your body and then straight up toward your face
- **Kicks**—bring your knee up then extend your leg straight out from your knee

)209(Shoot some hoops

If you live within a house or two of a man (any man!) chances are there's a basketball hoop nearby. Get a ball and start shooting away. No net? Grab a ball and just play catch with yourself (or someone else). You'll work torso muscles you haven't felt since sixth grade gym class and you'll burn those calories even if you don't score!

)210(Go for a spin!

Bicycling is a great calorie burner, whether you're on a stationary cycle or heading around the block. Plus, once again, your ab muscles will be engaged as you move your legs.

)211(Play the field

Just get outside! Run around your lawn, sprint, play hopscotch, do cartwheels, practice skipping! Sound crazy? Playing like this will burn almost 90 calories and it will improve your mood because it's nothing but fun.

)212(Practice your swing

Got a golf club or a baseball bat? Start swinging—the twisting motion is great not only for your obliques (the side ab muscles), but also your for you core muscles, which keep your middle flat and toned.

)213(Carry a big heavy load up a hill

Now, this may sound silly, but I thought you might want to know that combining extra weight, going uphill, and walking is perhaps the number one way to burn huge numbers of calories. That's right! In just 10 minutes you'll take off a whopping 90 calories. Not in the mood to strap a load on and climb a mountain? Carry your groceries up the stairs.

)214(Jump in!

I realize it's not that easy to swim for just 10 minutes, but, truth be told, some women can't swim for much longer than that if they've just started working out. And, if you're sitting by the pool on a hot day, what's so wrong with jumping in every now and then?

)215(Rake the leaves

Okay, this one is seasonal too, but I just thought I'd let you know that the rake is your friend. The back and forth motion will force your abs to work. Chiropractors advise switching sides often to prevent strain which will also help work the obliques on both sides.

)216(Scrub

Look at your bathroom. Do you give it due respect? How about your kitchen floor? Mopping a floor or scrubbing a shower is a great way to burn calories, strengthen your muscles (abs and arms), and take care of yourself (well, your home).

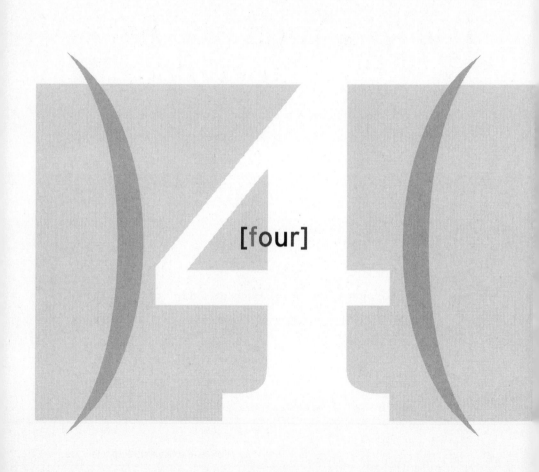

[four]

The Get Your Abs Back After Pregnancy Plan

It's a paradox: The moment you need your abs to be stronger and more centered than ever—to help you pick up your infant, muscle that heavy diaper bag, and wrestle the stroller into the trunk—is when they're at their weakest. Getting your abdominal muscles back in shape after delivery is essential for helping you make it through baby boot camp without painful back injuries or feeling overloaded by the task of getting through the day carrying around (and getting up and down with) an 8 to 20 pound (or more) baby all day long. Not to mention that it'd be nice to lose the jiggle around your middle. With your doctor's okay, many new mothers resume their exercise program a couple of weeks after delivery. Of course, C-section moms need to wait longer. Discuss your exercise plans with your doctor and take it slow. Throughout pregnancy, there's also plenty you can do to keep your ab muscles strong to prevent the low back aches so common during pregnancy and to help give you needed strength during labor. Talk to your doctor about your workout beforehand and listen to any advice about exercises you should avoid, especially if you have a high risk pregnancy. ~

)217(Stretch your abdomen

Kneel on the ground with your torso erect. Reach your arms around your back as far as you can with your fingertips pointing downward. Press your hips forward and pivot your shoulders back to feel the stretch. Try this move before an ab workout or anytime your core feels stressed and fatigue.

)218(Let your clothes cling

Look for the latest styles made of trendy, clingy fabrics that contour your curves and even give a flash of your belly. These body-hugging fabrics flatter your pregnant shape more than oversized t-shirts and sweaters.

workbook

)219(Did you know?

Eating healthy and doing some toning exercises will help you cope with the third trimester aches and speed your efforts to get your body back after pregnancy. In fact, the American College of Obstetrics and Gynecology advises pregnant and postpartum women to engage in 30 minutes or more of moderate exercise on most, if not all, days of the week. In many cases, you can continue your vigorous pre-pregnancy exercise program. However, if the thought of getting down to the floor conjures up fears of not being able to get back up, don't worry. Ab work can be modified during pregnancy to make exercising for two possible. The exercises shouldn't cause discomfort to your belly or your back. To be safe, always consult your obstetrician before trying any exercise routine, especially if you are in a high risk pregnancy. If your doctor advises against crunches, listen. And as a general rule of thumb, avoid full crunches altogether and take the propped-up and sitting up exercises out of your program after the fifth month of pregnancy to ensure the inferior vena cava—a vein responsible for returning blood to the heart that the pregnant uterus presses against when lying on your back—does not get pinched and cause dizziness.

Warm up for three minutes with some light walking or stair-climbing and neck, torso, and leg stretches. Then try the exercises from this chapter that are appropriate for pregnancy and post-pregnancy tummy toning. Begin with fewer repetitions than you have done in the past and focus on proper form and maintaining a transverse abdominis contraction by exhaling completely on each breath throughout each session. If you can only do one rep, that's okay. One friend of mine swears she got her tummy back by doing one sit up just one day after her baby was born, and adding one more every day. By the end of two weeks, she could do 14 a day and stayed at that number for a few months to lose her baby weight.

)220(Cool an itchy belly

If you are experiencing an itchy belly, your skin may feel scratchy from all the stretching going on as collagen fibers expand to make room for the baby. Pregnancy is not the time to experiment with stretch mark treatments. But there are quick, safe ways to relieve an itchy belly:

- Try taking cooler showers as hot water can aggravate the rash.
- Moisturize.
- Do whatever you need to do to cool down.
- Pregnancy belly balms and oils are packed with emollient moisturizers that can ease itchiness from stretching skin.
- Over-the-counter itch creams can help. Get your health care provider's okay first.
- Try taking a soothing oatmeal bath and using sensitive skin products that are oatmeal based.

)221(Erase the mommy streak

Many women develop darkening or hyperpigmentation during pregnancy. One common spot is the called the *linea nigra*, where pigmentation of the skin spans from the belly button down to the pubic bone during pregnancy. It often disappears on its own, in time. If it doesn't, or you want to speed its disappearing act, over-the-counter cosmetic bleaching creams can help. They contain two percent hydroquinone to stop the production of melanin in the skin zone and to help lighten existing dark spots. Some may also contain fading ingredients such as kojic acid or azelaic acid. Never use them during pregnancy or breastfeeding. Apply the cream daily to clean, dry skin. If you don't see the results you want after several daily applications, see a dermatologist who can prescribe a prescription-strength formula which will contain a higher percentage of bleaching ingredient than can be sold in the cosmetics aisle.

)222(Get checked

If you experience symptoms such as abdominal pain, nausea, cramping, bloating, gas, and diarrhea after eating or drinking dairy, see your doctor and ask if you could be suffering from lactose intolerance. Milk products contain lactose, and during the digestion process an enzyme in your intestines breaks down lactose into smaller, more easily digested sugars. If you have lactose intolerance, your body produces too few lactase enzymes to break down dairy. If you think you're lactose intolerant, don't just give up dairy. See your doctor who can help you determine how much dairy your individual body can comfortably digest and help you come up with a plan for healthy eating.

) 223 (Slather on a firming lotion

Skin firming lotions help you achieve more toned, firmer skin. The makers of these creams back up their claims with clinical studies showing that the lotions help firm, tone, and soften skin in as little as two weeks. The latest firming lotions contain a variety of ingredients (Co-enzyme Q10, Biotin, and caffeine, to name a few) to help repair skin's elasticity, which naturally decreases with age. By helping repair the skin's collagen and elastin matrix, the skin appears younger and more taut. Smooth a skin firming lotion on your stomach one to two times per day to help tighten and tone. Avoid using during pregnancy or breast feeding without your doctor's okay.

)224(Massage to the rescue

There's nothing that feels better postpartum than a full body massage complete with lavender massage oil and a masseuse named Hans. Before your trip back to reality–diaper changes, burping baby, and mounting laundry–taking time to get yourself a massage can do wonders for your body and mind (and waistline).

• Massage therapy reduces water retention, helping eliminate any water-weight gain you may be experiencing.

• Massaging your abdomen in circular motions on a daily basis can help ease the cramping discomfort in the postpartum time period. Massage may also help your abdomen return to its pre-pregnancy shape through a process called uterine involution that encourages your uterus to contract and pass the postpartum discharge.

• While you may be focusing on losing all that extra baby weight, you're also watching the scale to make sure baby is gaining. Research shows simple infant massage can help stimulate infant weight gain.

• Stress can work against your weight loss efforts and when baby's on a crying jag or you're feeling generally overwhelmed with new motherhood, your stress levels can peak. Research shows infant massage improves the mother-infant interaction and lessens feelings of postnatal depression.

• Massage in general makes you feel better about yourself and your body, which can help maintain your interest in sticking to weight loss efforts to improve postpartum self-esteem.

• Massage can ease the back pain associated with pregnancy weight gain and infant care (lifting baby, diaper bags, and the stroller). It also helps soothe the aches and pains of the pregnancy, delivery, and postpartum periods.

• Gently massaging an area that's recently healed from a wound can minimize or even eliminate scarring. Massage can also even out a raised scar from a surgery (such as a C-section). Avoid touching the area early on when your body is still healing. Ask your doctor for the green light to try gentle massage at your six week checkup, once the wound has completely healed. Use a sweet almond, jojoba, or olive oil and gently press on the new scar making small, sweeping circular motions. You'll help break down scar tissue with your gentle strokes for a smoother appearance.

)225(Don't lie down after dinner

Lying down after a meal can cause excess gas and bloating to build and expand the abdomen. Ease digestion by standing or sitting—better yet, go for a walk to help your body process that meal more quickly.

)226(Solve constipation

If you look a little bloated in the lower abdomen, waste left in the intestines may be to blame. A "full" gastrointestinal track causes a bloated look, says nutritionist Cynthia Sass, RD, spokesperson for the American Dietetic Association. Whether your GI is full of air, gasses, carbonation, or waste, the fullness expands the contents of the intestines, which are all coiled up right there in the abdomen, giving you that "early pregnancy" look. Ask your doctor what remedies might be right for you.

)227(Press pause on cravings

Eat when you are hungry—your body needs the extra calories. Reach for healthy foods first (a bowl of broccoli, yogurt) and chances are that you won't have much of a taste for pickles and ice cream.

)228(Step off the scale

During pregnancy don't use your little passenger as an excuse to eat for an entire family. But you also shouldn't count calories obsessively either—let your doctor gauge your weight gain at your appointments.

Fitness Fun

)229(Chair raises or chair crunches

Sit on the edge of a chair so that your toes touch the floor and your knees are bent. Tighten your core muscles and balance yourself by grasping the sides of the chair seat on either side of you. Lean into the chair so that your shoulder blades are reclined against the chair back. Don't let your back curve. Inhale while lifting your right knee up toward your chest as high up as is comfortable. Exhale and do a gentle crunch with your knee lifted. Open your chest and lower your leg to the starting position with your toes on the floor. Repeat 8 to 15 reps with each leg.

)230(Single-leg toe taps

Lie on your back. Lift your legs to the ceiling and bend your knees so your legs are make a ninety-degree angle. When you first attempt this exercise, hang your heels close to your rear to relax your thigh muscles during this movement. Pull your belly button in and press your low back into the floor. Use your abs to maintain this spinal position as you move your legs. Breath in. Hold your breath as you lower one leg to the floor until the toes tap the floor, then exhale as you return the leg back to the beginning position. To challenge your abs more, if you are able to hold the spinal position, move your heel further and further away from your butt as you lower your toes.

)231(Propped-up sit ups

Stack four to six bed pillows or shams against a wall at a 45-degree angle. Sit down on the floor and lean up against the pillows, making sure you're comfortably supported and your head is several inches higher than your knees. Place your feet hip-width apart with your hands behind your head for support. Contract your stomach so your spine is in a neutral (non-curved) position. Inhale and lift your upper body off the pillows. Inhale and lower yourself. Be sure not to strain your neck by pulling on it with your hands. Do two sets of 8 to 12 reps (or less—gauge your own comfort level), being sure to rest as needed between sets.

)232(Tummy tuck-ins

Get on all fours so that your hands are shoulder-width apart and your knees are hip-width apart. Look at the floor about a foot in front of you so that your neck is straight—not raised or dropped. Tighten your abs for support and keep your back from sagging or humping—your spine and abs should both be in the neutral position. Take a breath. Exhale and pull your belly button up and in. Hold. Release. Do one to two sets of 8 reps, resting as needed between set.

workbook

)233(Did you know?

Not only can pregnancy and delivery stretch your tummy, you may also be suffering from urine loss. This is called stress urinary incontinence. One simple way to both tighten your abs and stop this embarrassing urine loss is to do Kegels (which, by the way, will help you enjoy sex again and achieve better orgasms in only a week's time).

Kegels involve contracting the muscles used to stop urinating. While you should never stop your urine when going to the bathroom because it can cause infection, take that information and practice shutting off your urine stream when you're not going. Practice while driving, showering, pushing the stroller, or nursing, until your muscles feel fatigued. Once you're good at Kegels, you can simultaneously tone your ab muscles and enhance the potency of this exercise by pulling your belly button up and in (like you're buttoning tight jeans).

)234(Prone tabletop posture

Get on your hands and knees and make your back as flat as a table. Extend your left leg behind you until it is parallel to the floor. Your hips should be flat (don't lift your hip when you extend your leg). Next, extend your right arm straight ahead of you until it is alongside your right ear. Hold this posture for 15 seconds. Make sure you are engaging your lower abdominals throughout this posture. Challenge yourself more by lifting your right calf off the ground so that only your knee is supporting you. Try this on both sides.

)235(Prone oblique contractions (external oblique)

Begin in the table position. Extend your right arm in front of you and your left leg behind you. Bend your left knee bring it in toward your chest. Rotate your ribs slightly to the left as you pull your right elbow across your left knee. You should feel the contraction of muscle on the right waist line. Hold for a beat and then return to the beginning position.

)236(Use a baby carrier

Baby carriers keep baby close and your arms free to do other things. They also keep baby correctly positioned to reduce back strain. In terms of weight loss, strapping baby on is equivalent to strapping on the weighted vests used as fitness equipment. You'll burn more calories toting baby and tone your entire core by engaging the ab and back muscles to stand up straight with baby's extra weight.

)237(Half sit ups

Sit straight up on the floor, bend your knees and stretch your arms out in front of you. Engage your abdominals by drawing your navel in toward your spine. Gently lean backwards and stay in this position for ten counts. Repeat up to 10 times.

)238(Weight gain is not your destiny

Research shows gaining weight after age 30 is due to lack of exercise and healthy eating habits as well as a depressed mood. If you fear getting older means automatically inheriting your Aunt Gertrude's inner tube, stay on top of your workout efforts and healthy eating habits. Exercise will also go a long way to boost mood-improving serotonin levels in your brain to help you keep a sleek physique.

Baby as Fitness Tool

Incorporate baby into your get-your-abs-back routine. Try these moves once baby has head control:

) **239** (Peek-a-boo crunches

Sit down on the floor, bend your knees, and put your feet flat on the floor. Take your baby and place him lying on your shins with his face peering just above your knees. Hold him securely on his sides and cross your feet. Gently roll backwards until you're lying flat on the floor and baby is resting on your shins. Tighten your abs and lift your head, neck, and shoulders off the ground, giving baby a big grin and "peek-a-boo" as you come up. Take a deep breath and return to start. Repeat. Gradually build up to two sets of 12 reps.

)240(Baby lifts

Stand with feet hip-width apart and your hips tilted slightly forward. Lean your shoulders back, engage your ab muscles and lift your chest slightly. Hold baby securely under the armpits in front of you at belly button level. Slowly raise baby (arms' length away) until your arms are slightly above shoulder height. Say, "Up-sey, girl" and watch her giggle.

)241(Airplane rides

Stand with your feet hip-width apart, and hips tilted slightly forward. Tighten your abs and lift your chest, shoulders dropped. Hold baby securely under the armpits in front of you at belly button level, facing you. Twist (without moving your hips—remember to stabilize your pelvis) side-to-side mimicking a "vroom, vroom" airplane sound.

Nutrition Nuggets

)242(Be patient

The pudge will budge, but not overnight. Dieting is never a good idea at this point, as you'll need the calories to keep up with infant care demands and to produce breast milk if you're breastfeeding. But do start scaling your portions back slightly so that you're not still eating your pre-delivery amount.

)243(Create colorful plates

Your meal should be centered around plenty of colorful vegetables (green, red, yellow) and low-fat proteins. Then, add whole grains to your meals. Fruit is great for dessert or a snack, but try to add a protein each time you eat fruit.

) 244 (Change the way you grocery shop

Nutritionists recommend shopping the perimeter of the store, hitting the fruits and vegetable aisle first, then pick up low-fat dairy products, lean ground sirloin or turkey and chicken, whole grain breads, fish, and frozen vegetables. Then travel around the inner aisles. If you're on a budget, total your initial items before adding in the processed food items found in the middle aisles that'll add heft to your grocery bill and your waistline.

) 245 (Lose white foods (except for cauliflower)

Eliminate simple carbohydrates or highly processed foods, such as white bread, white rice, and non-whole wheat pasta. White carbs spike blood sugar levels and cause cravings, causing you to eat more than you need.

)246(Did you know?

Water is something you need to think about when exercising—at home or

in the gym. A study from Gatorade showed that nearly half of all exercisers

are already dehydrated when they arrive at the gym. One could assume the

same thing goes for at-home exercisers who lace up their sneakers to do an

exercise video or go for a jog. By the time you feel thirsty, you're already

dehydrated. And just being slightly dehydrated—as little as two percent—can

negatively affect your endurance during exercise and make your muscles

fatigue faster. Exercise physiologists say the better hydrated you stay, the

better you feel, so you can exercise at a higher intensity for longer and burn

more calories. Water is also an important weight loss tool that helps flush

the body and helps fill you up to curb cravings and snacking.

As a general guideline, you need eight glasses of water per day. Guzzle 17 to 20 ounces within two hours before activity. During exercise, you also need to replace fluids you're losing through sweat. Take in 8 ounces every 15 minutes during exercise. Since it can be nearly impossible to keep track while drinking out of your water bottle, try this trick: Count gulps. Every gulp is about 1 ounce. So take 8 gulps every 15 minutes of exercise to replace fluid loss. Up your gulps if you're sweating more than usual. Squeeze some lemon or lime in your glass, add a splash of fruit juice, or try a sports drink to help you down your daily dose.

)247(Drink herbal tea

Chase your meal with a cup of peppermint or chamomile tea, which helps aid digestion and calms frayed nerves. The water will keep you hydrated and the herbs will support a good mood and a healthy stomach. Green tea is even said to burn fat!

)248(Drinking something with dinner?

Use small, Dixie-sized cups to get the right amount—$^3/_4$ cup is a serving size.

) 249 (Marinate your food

Marinate foods in the refrigerator for 24 hours before cooking to ensure they're saturated with mouth-watering flavor. For chicken, try a mixture of fresh lemon juice, lemon zest, onion, and rosemary. Combine orange juice, shallot, and dill for a delicious salmon marinade.

) 250 (Alter your pyramid

Instead of centering your meals around a starchy food, such as pasta, instead, plan your meals (including snacks) around two things: low-fat proteins and vegetables. Making sure each of your meals includes these two food types will insure that you most likely take in the proper nutrients throughout the day. Limiting the saturated fats that go along with the meal will help you get the right number of calories, too.

) 251 (Find new rewards

If a piece of chocolate (or an entire candy bar or a pint of ice cream) is your reward to yourself after a hard day (or any day) come up with a list of 10 alternative stress-relievers to give yourself a boost. Some ideas? A manicure, a new paperback novel, an at-home facial, or, how about a 10-minute yoga session!

workbook

)252(What exactly is a mini-meal?

Anything between 300 and 400 calories constitutes a mini-meal. Eating five or six of these a day (for a maximum total of 2400 calories) is far better than eating three 800-calorie meals. Your body digests the smaller numbers of calories much more easily.

Some suggestions:

- 1 chicken drumstick and an apple
- granola (including chocolate morsels and dried fruit) with yogurt
- 2 eggs with spinach and 1 slice of toast
- ¾ cup of high-fiber cereal with skim milk and an orange
- half a tuna sandwich with lettuce and tomato
- a big salad with a hard-boiled egg and 2 Tbsp dressing

)253(Hang forward

If gravity is working against you, you're not alone. A prominent personal trainer confirmed that breasts start to sag as early as the mid-twenties in most women. If you've had children, the effects are magnified sooner, especially if you've breastfed. If you're bothered by sagging breasts, hang forward while putting on your bra or swimsuit. Lift each breast up with a hand as you put on the bra to help them sit higher in the cups. Fasten and stand up. You'll get more cleavage and less droop. In addition to hanging forward, one celebrity stylist told me celebrities solve the problem with padded, seamless Wonderbras with a support system that make their breasts look perkier.

)254(Leave the string at home

Opt out of string bikinis and go for the tankini that will camouflage those last few pounds of baby weight you haven't quite lost yet.

)255(Wrap it up

Wrapped tops and skirts are particularly flattering for the pregnant body.

Pregnancy and Post-Pregancy Dos and Don'ts

)256(DON'T do these activities

Obstetricians caution against activities that could cause abdominal trauma such as ice hockey, kickboxing, soccer, and horseback riding.

)257(DON'T try any new exercise routine without your doctor's okay

This is especially important if you have experienced risk factors, such as vaginal bleeding.

)258(DON'T keep exercising

If you feel dizzy, faint, overheated, or nauseous, stop and call your doctor.

)259(DON'T do back-lying exercises for more than three minutes

Back-lying exercises after the fourth month of your pregnancy must be modified because in this position the uterus can press on the vena cava, which runs down the right side of the body.

)260(DON'T complete the recommended number of reps

If you feel any pain or discomfort or if something just doesn't feel right, stop immediately.

)261(DON'T expect to resume your pre-pregnancy workout

Give yourself several weeks to gradually work back up to your previous fitness level. Start slowly at first after your doctor gives you the green light to go ahead and begin exercising again following delivery.

)262(DO bring baby along

After baby's born, instead of trying to separate from baby and juggle feedings, naps, a babysitter, and your workout schedule, try bringing baby along in a stroller or in a baby carrier. Try Mommy-and-Me exercise classes that involve playing with baby as part of the exercise routine. You'll also be sending your child an important message that exercise is healthy and important to living a good life.

)263(Dress sexy

If you're feeling fat rather than pregnant, the solution may be baring your belly. The burgeoning pregnant belly has a sexy curve. And oversized clothes do have a way of draping and making you feel like you're a plus, plus size. Don't be afraid of cute belly-baring, body-hugging clothes during pregnancy.

)264(Drawstring power

Drawstring pants are your friend. The dangling string visually creates a diagonal line to slim your shape.

Post-Pregnancy Waistline Whittling Exercises

You shake your head side to side every time you undress and see that extra inch on either side of your waistband. Now it's time to twist your torso doing exercises that'll shrink your sides. You've probably crunched yourself silly trying to undo the extra padding around your waistline, to no avail. Twisting is the only motion that engages the obliques, the long muscles responsible for sideways motions that run diagonally up the sides, from the pelvis to the ribs. So if you want to break up with your love handles or prevent them from ever joining your sleek physique, do twisting exercises approximately three (non-consecutive) days a week. Twisters help strengthen the back too, improving your posture with the important balance of both strong abs and back.

)265(Torso twisters

Sit with your feet flat on the floor, hip-width apart. Clasp your hands with your arms outstretched. Lower yourself to a 45-degree angle, contracting your abs for support. Twist your arms and upper body to the right. Return to center. Now twist to the left. Do 8 to 15 reps per side. For more of a challenge, hold each position (right, center, left) for 10 counts. Lie back onto the floor and hug your knees into your chest to release your muscles.

)266(Straight leg twist ups

Lie on your back, left leg bent and foot flat on the floor. Stretch your right leg out, resting it on the floor. Place your right arm across your waist and your left hand behind your head. Twist up, bringing the left elbow to the right knee. Switch sides. Do two sets of 15 to 25 reps.

)267(Cross twist ups

Lie on the floor as though you're going to do crunches: Bend your knees, feet flat on the floor, hands supporting the back of your head. Inhale and lift your head and upper shoulders off the ground and reach your right elbow to your left knee as you simultaneously lift the knee up toward the elbow. Return to start. Repeat with the left elbow and right knee. Do 8 to 12 reps.

)268(Bicycles

To up the ante on the previous exercise, hold your feet up off the floor in the starting position. Put both hands behind your head. Bring your right elbow up toward the bent left knee, then, while still holding your crunch position, switch sides. Straighten your left leg, twist up your left elbow and bring in your right knee to meet it. Continue switching sides, bicycling your legs, 15 to 25 times

)269(Side planks

Lie on your right side with knees bent, resting your upper body on your elbow. Lift your body as far off the floor as you can, and hold for 10 seconds. Repeat on the other side.

)270(Put up your dukes

The cross-body motion of boxing shapes the waist and helps knock out stress. Make fists, twist, and jab, then twist and punch in the other direction. Do 60.

)271(Replace your desk chair with a Fitball

This will force you to sit up straight, and strengthen both your abs and legs.

)272(Upward side twists

Lie on your stomach on the floor with your feet together and arms under your shoulders with your upper body weight supported on your elbows and forearms. Lift and partly rotate your upper body toward the right, lifting your right elbow to point to 10 o'clock while balancing your weight on your left elbow and hip. Keep your feet on the floor. Return to the start and repeat on the other side. Do one set of 16 reps.

)273(Oblique twists

Sit on the floor and lean back about 45 degrees while holding a 5-pound dumbbell with both hands (dumbbell optional). Keep your belly button firmly pulled into your spine. Now slowly twist from side to side while contracting the abdominal area. Do two sets of 25 reps (one rotation right and left equals one rep).

) 274 (Leg twists

Lie on your back, bent knees, feet on the floor. Raise your upper body
into a crunch, with your hands behind your head. Lift your legs so your
toes rest on the ground. Drop the knees to the right side, then center, then
left. Pivot your legs on your toes, making a pendulum motion. Do two sets
of 8 to 15.

) 275 (Side twists

Begin kneeling, and lean over, placing your right hand on the floor.
Extend your left leg out, lift your left hand toward the sky, and gaze
upward. Tighten your torso and reach your left arm through the open
space between your supporting arm and leg. Keep your hips up and do
5 reps on each side.

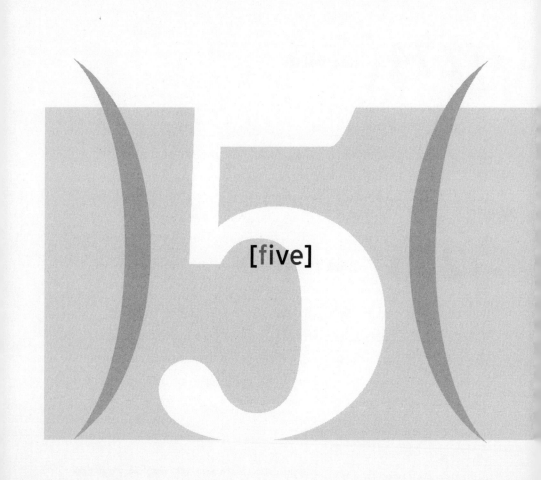

[five]

The Bikini Beach Plan

Ah, the beach. There are few fashion dreams as ubiquitous as a woman strolling down the beach in a string bikini. But most of us never really do just that. Anyone can, though. All it takes is a little effort and a lot of confidence! ~

Health and Beauty Bytes

) 276 (Get a shimmery glow

By now, everyone knows the fun has been taken out of sun. But you can banish the unbaked cookie dough look simply by slathering on one of the new generation of body highlighters, body oil mists, or self-tanners. They can all add definition and sex appeal to your mid-region—and the results are only a slather away..

) 277 (Get auto-bronzed

Book a spa appointment for a professional airbrushed and streak-less faux tan (about $100 and up for 45 minutes). Opt for airbrushing done by a spa technician or a booth. Hollywood celebrities used to get self-tanned by their makeup artists for films. Now makeup artists say they send their movie stars straight to the auto-bronzing booth for an all-over tan. Auto-bronzing is quite quick in the booth, but some prefer the accuracy of a professional bronzing. In either case, it'll take you no more than an hour to complete the process, from booking to a total tan.

)278(Feeling misty

Featherweight, water-based spray moisturizers mist onto skin for quick application and a subtle sheen. Body-oil sprays are a little greasier, but they deliver in the shine department. For softer, smoother skin, try misting your middle immediately after your shower while your skin is still damp to lock in moisture droplets. A light sheen will remain and add a dash of shimmer to your midsection.

workbook

Give yourself just the right all-over color

If you want a tropical look for under $30, self-tanning is for you. A faux glow makes you look thinner, healthier, and visually lengthens your ab muscles and limbs. A bronzed tan even conceals cellulite and other skin imperfections like scars and stretch marks. Self-tanners give an all-over foundation of color for anytime. Today's self-tanners have a chemical in them that gradually—and safely—darken the skin without turning you an Agent Orange hue. Plus, it's a whole lot safer than exposing your skin to harmful UVA and UVB rays. Dermatologists give them the nod, saying color from a tube gives the look of spending two weeks in Aruba without putting your skin at risk. While UV damage from a real tan puts you at risk for sunspots, hyperpigmentation, and skin cancer, there are no side effects with a fake tan (unless you do a sloppy job).

While slathering on a self-tanner takes 30 minutes, you'll need to spend a few minutes prepping yourself. Here's how.

)279(Pick your hue

What's in: a hint of color. *What's out:* a deep bronzed look. Choose shades based on your actual skin tone, not a tropical color. If you're fair skinned, go with light formulas for a honey hue instead of trying to look deeply-baked. If you're olive-skinned, try slightly darker tones. For believable results, use a different shade for your face and body.

)280(Choose your formula

Self-tanners come in sprays (great for reaching your back), lotions, foams, and gels. Choose the consistency you like working with best—do you like the feel of gel, the playfulness of foam, or the familiarity of lotion? Tinted self-tanners are helpful because they allow you to see where you've applied and where you've missed and give instant color.

)281(Test the tone

Check out the formula before you make a whole-body mistake. Do a spot test on the inside of your wrist—just open the tube and swipe some on. Wait an hour for the results.

)282(Exfoliate first

For an even, flawless finish, try a manual exfoliator such as a sugar scrub, body puff, or body polish. Use in the morning as part of your shower and plan to self-tan before bed.

)283(Streak-free sun swiping

• For smoother application and palms that aren't tanned, wear latex gloves (available at most drugstores).

• Your skin should be clean and dry. Apply body lotion only to the center of your stomach up to your chest before applying self-tanner. This is a celebrity makeup artist trick to help you look thinner. When you apply your self-tanner, the lotion will create a contrast, keeping the center of your stomach lighter than the sides. As a result, your obliques will be darker than the center of your stomach, making your abs look totally toned. The effect is thinning.

)284(Start Tanning

• Squeeze out a quarter-sized dollop of self-tanner. Use long, even strokes to apply. Work from top to bottom. Massage therapists are usually the ones doing self-tanner application at the salon, so try to mimic long effleurage motions rather than smearing it on.

• Apply the tanner lightly and evenly, rubbing well into the skin.

• Go light on your elbows, knees, and feet—these callused areas grab more tanner and end up darker than the rest of you.

- Tanners tend to accentuate freckles, hyperpigmentation (such as the *linea nigra*, a darkened line from the belly button down to the pelvis bone that develops during pregnancy in some women), beauty marks, and liver spots. To prevent this, apply a little petroleum jelly to the spot so the tanner cannot be absorbed there.

- After application, let the tanner dry a few minutes, then buff yourself all over. To ensure evenness, use an old athletic sock turned inside out so the terry is rubbing the skin. Move the terry mitt in small circular motions, working from top to bottom to prevent lines and streaks.

- Practice on your legs first to master the art of achieving even, all-over color.

- Don't forget your navel. Apply a small amount inside your belly button. Be sure to go back with a dry cotton swab to remove any excess. Otherwise you'll end up with a belly button that's darker in the interior folds, which will make it look dirty inside.

- Stay nude for as long as you can—at least 10 to 15 minutes—to let the formula dry before putting on clothing.
- Wear old underwear and darkly colored clothes in case the formula stains. Tanning action happens gradually for several hours after application, so slip into loose, non-silk clothing that won't rub off the formula when you get dressed.
- To maintain your gorgeous golden glow, reapply self-tanner every two to three days.

)285(Go minty

Peppermint is a hot ingredient for many belly-loving lotions and potions. This cool, refreshing scent is great for hot days, as the actual minty-fresh action helps (very slightly) lower your body temperature.

)286(Banish a boring bikini line

Instead of making the commitment to a real tattoo, spas are starting to offer semi-permanent tattoos that last for two weeks and look like the real thing, without the permanency of a real tattoo. Artists at the hip Completely Bare Salon in NYC use a henna leaf paste solution to create a semi-permanent tattoo for $105. A Mendhi artist creates the tattoo and uses crystals to highlight the vibrant design. Place one just below your belly button or right below the waistband of your low-slug jeans so that it peaks out slightly for a sexy look.

workbook

)287(Did you know?

A fake tan does not protect you from sunburn. While you might not think about slathering your stomach with sunscreen before going outside when wearing midriff-baring tops and low-slung jeans, it's worth the effort. Your tummy skin is susceptible to burns just like everywhere else. Be sure to screen before heading out. Not only is a burned belly less than flattering, it's very uncomfortable when you sit, stand, or bend. If you get burned, try aloe vera gel. Or make a cup of black tea and let it steep and cool. Tea contains bioflavonoids, which are plant compounds with anti-inflammatory properties. Use the tea bags to dab cool tea on the sunburn for an instant *ahhh*. And be sure you pass on Mexican food when sunburned because hot and spicy foods will make your blood vessels dilate and make you look even redder.

Tanning Dos and Don'ts

) 288 (DO wait twenty minutes

Ater showering, bathing, or swimming you should wait twenty minutes before tanning for best results. In a hurry? Dry off well and use a hair dryer to speed-dry damp spots.

) 289 (DON'T shave that day

Razors tend to rough up the area around the follicles, causing tanner to absorb in a polka-dot pattern. Avoid shaving immediately after self-tanning, as it will remove color.

)290(DON'T use a self-tanner before laser hair removal

A faux glow decreases the laser beam's effectiveness.

)291(DO wear gloves

You don't want unnatural looking tanned palms!

)292(DO avoid tanning your arches

This is a dead giveaway that you didn't just vacation in the Caribbean.

)293(DON'T use moisturizer

You need to let the tanner do its work for at least a half an hour.

)294(DO avoid getting wet

No showering or swimming, or working up a sweat at the gym for 12 hours after application. One woman ruined a $125 professional tan when her dog licked her just-bronzed leg.

)295(DO pick the color you would naturally tan

Don't pick a bronze that is too dark or anything that seems somewhat orange.

)296(Minimize hair's reappearing act

Dermatologists can prescribe Vaniqua, which helps inhibit hair growth. Over the counter versions by Curel and Jegens are available as well.

)297(Blonde your body hair

If you have sparse body hair but wish it were lighter, a new Brazilian treatment available at spas gives the whole body a salt scrub and bleach treatment. This is different than bleaching your tummy track at home. Applied from head to toe, the salt smoothes and exfoliates the skin for a softer, sleeker appearance, while the bleach lightens each and every body hair to a pale, golden yellow. With all of your body hair turned blonde, you'll be able to bare your midriff without feeling self-conscious about dark body hair.

workbook

)298(Remove the fuzz

Whisk away that treasure trail. When wearing midriff-baring clothes or a bathing suit, get in the habit of always inspecting your below-the-belly-button zone for wayward hairs . Look yourself over in a well-lit room near a sunlit window. Here are some de-fuzzing options, which vary in price and potency. The same methods can also be used to clean up your bikini line.

)299(Shaving

Shaving is not an ideal method for cleaning your bikini zone, as you will get stubble, but it is an easy once- or twice-a-week option. Make sure you lather up with a shave gel first, and replace your razor regularly to ensure it won't irritate the delicate bikini zone. Try a mini-razor sized for clearing this area of hair. OB/GYNs report a surge of women in their twenties and thirties shaving it all off for a smoother line in a bikini—bye, bye pelvic bulge. Shaving down under is best done with a mini razor or the new electric bikini trimmers, which work so much better than nail scissors or sewing shears to smooth the down-under zone.

Cost: $5, Zero ouches, unless you get nicked

)300(Salon

You can get a bikini line wax; a full Brazilian wax, which removes all pubic hair from the pubic bone back; or leave just a small "landing strip" or triangle of hair. Some spas offer signature waxes to shape the pubic hairs into Gucci "Gs" or Chanel "Cs" or whatever signature letter you choose.

Cost: At a salon: $40 for bikini wax, $50 for a Brazilian wax,

$10 for a tummy wax * Three ouches for a tummy wax,**

***** five ouches for the full Brazilian wax**

)301(Tweezing

This method is best for a few rogue, near-the-navel hairs that crop up every so often, but not for larger areas. Get yourself a precise pair of stainless steel, professional-grade tweezers like Tweezerman's that are precise enough to grab hold of escape-artist fine hairs. Use them in a pinch, or to clean up a stubborn hair or two missed during waxing.

Cost: $18 ** Two ouches

)302(Depilatory creams

A chemical cream you smooth on and wipe off that dissolves hair is fine for the bikini line, belly hair, and removing pubic hair (the pelvic bulge). Test on your inner arms a day in advance to check for irritation before use. The major drawback to this method is that depilatories have a strong odor. Choose ones with hair-growth inhibitors, such as fruit enzymes, that will encourage the hair to grow back finer and more

sparsely with every use.

Cost: about $7 * One ouch for sensitive skin

) 303 (Bleaching

Unless you really only have a couple of dark hairs, bleaching is not an

ideal method for belly fuzz but can be useful for other areas with hair.

When the light hits your belly in a certain way, everyone will see the thick

track of golden blonde hair you're sporting. Smooth is better, so go for a

method that leaves your skin perfectly hair-free.

Cost: about $6 to bleach belly hair at home,

$120 for Brazilian bleaching and exfoliation

* One ouch for sensitive skin

)304(Waxing or sugaring

Hot wax or sugaring products (made from sugar or honey instead of wax) adhere to the hairs and harden. When pulled off, they remove hair at the root. The sensation is similar to ripping off a gummy bandage. The skin may look pinkish for a little while afterward. The resulting smoothness can last from two to six weeks, depending on your hair growth. Contrary to common myth, your hair won't grow back thicker or courser. If anything, you'll see less hair and finer hair as follicles become damaged and no longer produce hair.

Bikini waxes can be done at home by sitting on a stool in a well-lit bathroom. Another, less messy option than dealing with a tub of hot wax at home are cold wax strips. These cellophane strips come pre-treated with wax and are suitable for the belly or face, but can't handle courser down-yonder hair. For better tugging power, warm the wax strips by cupping them in your hands and rubbing them vigorously. Peel and press the sticky side of the strip vertically onto your skin. Pull up and back quickly in the opposite direction of hair growth while holding the skin taut with your other hand. Remove any stickiness left on your stomach or bikini line with a little massage oil or baby oil. Redness should go away within 20 minutes or less, depending on how sensitive your skin is. Keep a couple of wax strips in your purse for an emergency ab clean up when changing into an outfit that will flash your midline for an after-work date.

Cost: $6 to 40 for an at-home kit   ***Three ouches

)305(Laser

Zapping your tummy hair-free is an option if you have black, brown, or dark blonde hair. Laser hair removal ranked as the fourth most common surgical cosmetic surgery procedure for women in 2002, according to The American Society for Aesthetic Plastic Surgery. Laser hair removal works best for those with light skin and dark hair because the laser is attracted to pigment in the hair and then travels into the follicle to destroy the strand at the root. Not even dying the hair would fool the beam. If you have dark skin and hair, you may experience hyperpigmentation (dark spots on the skin), so consider another option. It can take three, five, or more treatments to rid your belly of hair for good. For best results, avoid plucking, waxing, or shaving before a laser or pulsed light (similar to laser but uses infrared light) treatment.

Cost: $250 to $800 per treatment   * One ouch

)306(Electrolysis

This procedure is permanent and works on all skin and hair colors. However, it can take many sessions to achieve results. Electrolysis involves inserting a tiny needle into the natural opening of a follicle and releasing either a radio wave (a technique called thermolysis), a small electric galvanic current (traditional electrolysis), or a combination of the two methods to destroy the hair follicle. The number of sessions required to achieve permanent hair removal varies per person, but the bikini line can take over a year of treatment—requiring a total of 8-16 hours worth of treatment.

Cost: $30 to $85 per 15 to 30 minute session

*** Three ouches

)307(Fade stretch marks

Silvery white and pinkish colored marks are commonly found in areas such as the tummy, thighs, or breasts where the skin has been stretched due to pregnancy, rapid weight gain or growth (i.e. during adolescence), or elevated hormone levels. Dermatologists say the collagen-regenerating ingredient Vitamin A found in prescription Retin A and over-the-counter alpha hydroxy acids seems to diminish the appearance of some stretch marks when applied daily. Or, doctors can use a laser to remove stubborn marks with a flash of light. The laser light beam is passed over the stretch mark and converts the top superficial layers of skin into vapor, brushing away stretch marks for good. Cost: about $1,500 and up.

workbook

)308(Did you know?

OB/GYNs are reporting that shaving down below makes microscopic breaks in the skin, which make you slightly more susceptible to infections from hot tubs and STDs. Waxing may be a better option since it doesn't nick the skin.

)309(Take a good picture

Many of us suck in our guts when someone points a camera our way, but to look more natural (and yet slim), take a deep breath and then exhale, keeping your shoulders down and your belly in. Your abs will appear flat and your torso long.

Tummy trends

Several other ab trends take a little longer, but if you desire the abs of the moment, you may want to invest the time to see long-term results. Still, I think you're better off tightening and toning your abs for a sexier stomach with the shortcuts mentioned in earlier chapters than just scheduling a tummy tuck. And I think long, lean muscles in the abdomen are sexier by far than a belly button piercing. For my part, I wouldn't ever consider a tattoo or pierce. These trends aren't for everyone. But some trends are hard to ignore.

)310(Piercing and tattooing

Tattoos and navel piercing have been practiced for centuries. Ancient Egyptian pharaohs long ago practiced body art, piercing their navels during ceremonies as rites of passage. And many cultures, such as the Maori in New Zealand, have made great use of body art and tattoos. When considering a tattoo or navel pierce, be sure to consider your safety first. Tattoos are created by a small needle injecting ink into the dermal layer of the skin to create a permanent design. A small tattoo takes about 45 minutes and larger ones can take much longer, requiring repeat visits. It's also important to know that a tattoo can mask a melanoma on the skin's surface that would blend into the dye, preventing you or your doctor from ever seeing this warning sign of skin cancer before it's too late.

Piercing is invasive. It involves puncturing the skin with a needle and inserting a piece of jewelry into the opening. You should never try to do your own navel piercing because of risks of infection as well as the potential of misplacing a piercing or not placing it deep enough, which could result in the piercing being rejected by the body. Both piercing and tattooing expose you to the risks of allergic reactions, scar (keloid) formation, infection, and potential for exposure to diseases that are transmitted by needles.

If you do choose to get tattooed or pierced, choose a reputable place—in most states, body art studios are not regulated by state health departments, so the safety and cleanliness of establishments may vary. It's up to you to protect yourself by finding a body art salon that uses sanitary practices and can provide you with referrals. When visiting a body art studio for a tattoo or pierce, make sure you:

• Know your practitioner. Find a reputable piercing or tattoo studio with a well-trained staff.

- Ask for references.
- Look for cleanliness. Evaluate if there is an autoclave to sterilize equipment and observe if equipment is autoclaved between each use.
- Check that the technicians use gloves and change them before new procedures.
- Needles should be sterile and single use. Make sure the needle is unwrapped in front of you.
- Inks should never be reused.
- See your doctor or health care provider if you experience discomfort or infection (odorous, discolored discharge) after your piercing.

)311(Get to it sooner

New or "pink" stretch marks are easier to erase than older "white"
ones. Two at-home creams seem to help reduce the redness and ridging of
stretch marks. Check out Stretchaway from dermatologist Jeff Rapaport,
M.D. (call 800-951-3100) or Mustela 9 Months Stretch Marks Intensive
Action with herbal extracts (www.mustela.com). If you are seeking to
remove post-pregnancy stretch marks, wait until after delivery and breast
feeding to begin treatment. Many women swear by cocoa butter, although
there's been no clinical evidence that using it during pregnancy will keep
stretch marks at bay. However, giving this natural answer a try can't hurt.

)312(Reshaping the belly button

About fifteen percent of the population have "outies," according to Manhattan celebrity plastic surgeon Bruce Nadler, M.D. Being part of the "in" crowd is possible with a procedure called Umbilicoplasty, a two-hour outpatient surgery that runs from $3500 to over $5000. Even those with "innies" are booking belly button makeovers—special cosmetic lifts to elongate the navel and the look of the entire abdomen.

)313(Tummy tucking

Tummy tucking (abdominoplasty) involves removing excess flesh and tightening the belly. There are two basic types of tummy tuck procedures: the mini and modified tucks and the full abdominoplasty. The mini or modified tuck is preferable for those who have a stubborn fatty area below the belly button, but have good skin tone. This procedure involves a small, vertical incision (like a C-section) right above the pubic bone. The full abdominoplasty works best for those whose abdominal walls have been stretched by having children and whose skin and muscle tone is compromised. The physician may need to make an incision around the navel to help remove excess skin in this area. This procedure can also involve tightening the underlying abdominal muscles with sutures. Before you consider this procedure, make sure you're done having children. Otherwise, the effects will be undone.

Be sure to find a qualified plastic surgeon who is licensed and board certified. Ask for references and an interview before undergoing treatment. Also discuss with your surgeon before a procedure:

• Your medical history, including past and current medications and any existing or previous health problems.

• Surgical benefits, risks, and alternatives.

• Total cost, including surgeon, anesthesia, facility, and other fees.

Discuss the surgeon's policy on reversionary procedures as well as postsurgical care and the typical timeline for recovery.

workbook

Plastic Surgery Dos and Don'ts

)314(DO try diet and exercise first

Plastic surgery should be the last option!

)315(DON'T get caught up in a trend

Before you try a trendy new tummy tuck, be sure this is something you're willing to live with even when trends change. Consider your health, budget, and body image before making your decision. Be sure you're trying this fad because it's something you and you alone want—not something a partner or friend is pressuring you to try. Also invest time into finding the right expert to carry out your procedure—someone with a track record for doing exceptional work.

)316(DO search for the right facility

Do your homework to ensure you choose the right doctor (for plastic
surgery procedures) or body artists. References are a good way to locate
potential candidates, but also visit the facility, observe practices, and
ask questions.

)317(Did you know?

Several types of lasers can effectively remove tattoos. And unlike earlier procedures for tattoo removal, such as surgical removal or dermabrasion (course sanding of the skin), lasers are the most non-invasive way to undo a tattoo. Dermatologists can perform the procedure. In general, black and blue tattoos are the easiest to remove, while yellow and green colors are the most stubborn. The procedure involves treating the area with topical or local anesthesia and then passing a highly-concentrated laser beam over the area to vaporize the pigments. There are drawbacks: The process is painful, costly, and can result in scarring. Another procedure, laser ablation, involves the use of multiple lasers individually tuned to the various pigments to be removed. Although multiple sessions are necessary, this laser procedure is said to result in the least scarring.

Fitness Fun

) 318 (Beach ball crunches

Sit on a stability ball and recline so that the ball is under your back
and your feet are on the floor for support. Cross arms and lift into
a crunch. Do two sets of 10-15 reps. You can make it more of a
challenge by moving your feet closer together on the floor.

) 319 (Cardio abs

Try cardio classes that use a lot of side-to-side action to help activate
your ab muscles. Play basketball, swim, or take a kickboxing class.

) 320 (Tighten your torso

Lie on your back with a dumbbell in your left hand. Extend your arm on the floor at shoulder height. Rest your right arm at your side. Bend your left knee and place your foot on the floor. Extend your right leg out straight at a slight angle off the floor. Exhale, tighten your abs, and bring your left hand with the weight toward your right foot. Return to start. Do two sets of 12 to 15 reps, switching sides between sets.

) 321 (Plié

Sign up for a ballet class at your local health club. Unlike the formal ballet classes of your youth, these focus more on strength and stretching than grace alone. With the scales and tutus removed from the class, revisiting the willowy motions may add the missing component to your workout routine that'll help your flexibility and posture.

Nutrition Nuggets

)322(Don't starve yourself

Eat five to six small meals instead of three big ones. Research shows the human body burns calories more effectively when food consumption is spread out over the course of a day. Eating many small meals will also keep you from feeling hungry and gorging on too much food at one sitting—which forces the body to store the extra calories as fat.

)323(Help your muscles

Feed your muscles with healthy, low-fat protein sources. The protein will help give you a blast of sustained energy and make you feel fuller longer than carbohydrate snacks that leave you needing to refuel sooner and come loaded with salt (which makes you retain water).

workbook

Be a smart mouth

In an instant, you've raided the cupboards and devoured the chocolate chips, Oreos, and ice cream. To avoid stress snacking and letting your mouth take over all reason, follow these tips.

)324(DON'T buy it to begin with

Leave snack foods at the grocery store. Experts say one of the smartest ways to beat cravings is to not buy tempting foods to begin with.

)325(Try water

Sometimes the hunger cue is really thirst. Down 8 ounces of H_2O, which may wash away your urge to splurge.

)326(Have healthy food handy

Keep healthy snack foods readily available. If you've got your favorite good-for-you foods right on hand, you can appease those munchies without feeling guilty.

)327(Try visualization

Close your eyes and meet the ideal you—what size is she? Does she make strong and healthy eating choices? How does she keep her long-term goals in mind to resist passing cravings? Take a moment to do guided imagery to give you strength to work toward being the person you want to be.

)328(Drink through a straw

I know you're not drinking soda (too many bubbles that can bloat your belly), but in any case, a straw can help you to gulp less air.

)329(Enter the commercial-free zone

Studies show that seeing food can release a feel-good brain chemical called dopamine that can instantly trigger food cravings. Restaurant and snack food commercials on TV can be like a siren, calling you to the fridge to wreck your healthy eating habits. Walk away from the tube during commercial breaks or try doing some crunches (facing away from the TV), jumping jacks, or side twists. Exercise helps send cravings packing by waking up the satiety center of the brain.

) 330 (Manage monthly munchies

Studies show that cravings are particularly intense before menstruation. You may hit the carbs as a way to raise your brain's mood-boosting serotonin levels to counter PMS symptoms. Better: Drink a glass of skim milk, and feel free to pour in the fat-free chocolate sauce. You'll get a chocolate craving fix, plus calcium has been shown to help minimize PMS symptoms.

) 331 (Drink like a kid

You know those small plastic cups people use at barbecues and parties? Guess what: Fill that two-thirds of the way up and you've got yourself a serving of most beverages, such as wine, soda, and sports drinks. Use a small cup like that, rather than a large drinking glass, and you'll be sure to lose weight over time, as most of us drink twice that amount with meals.

)332(Shop in a farmer's market

Spend time shopping for fresh produce with a lot of zing: lemons, limes, blackberries, blueberries, mango, pineapple, red pepper, tomatoes, mesclun, garlic, green onions, and shallots.

The Look Great in a Bikini Workout

Pilates is the ultimate ab workout. Spend three minutes warming up and three minutes stretching. Round off the workout with a three minute cool down and finish with meditation.

)333(The hundred

Lie on your back and raise your legs to a 90-degree angle with your knees bent, arms at your sides. Tighten your abs and lift your head, neck, shoulders, and arms off the ground. Hold and start pumping your palms toward the ground in small patting motions. Inhale for a count of five and then exhale for five. Work up to ten sets of 10.

) 334 (The plank

Lie on your stomach with your forearms bent underneath you. Using your core muscles, lift your body upwards, balancing yourself on your forearms and toes with a flat back "plank" position. Hold for three counts. Do three sets of 5 reps.

) 335 (Leg circles

Lie on your back with your legs straight. Raise your right leg skyward and draw very small circles in the air with your toes pointed. Do five circles in one direction and then five in the reverse direction. Switch legs and repeat.

)336(Double leg stretch

Lie on your back, tuck in your chin and raise your head, arms and legs skyward. Sweep your arms outward and down along your sides and hug both knees to chest. Hold. Repeat 6 to 8 times.

)337(Rolling like a ball

Sit on the ground with knees bent and feet off the ground. Very lightly place hands on the tops of your shins. Round your back, tighten your abs and slowly roll backwards until your shoulder blades touch the ground. To perform this move properly, it is crucial for you to use your ab mucles to roll up, not the momentum from your legs. Repeat.

[acknowledgments]

This book would not have been possible without the hundreds of hours of interviews that sources have given me so generously over the last 10 years of my career. During that time period, many experts too numerous to list by name have assisted my reporting and understanding of dermatology, nutrition, fitness, health, and well-being. This book results from their time and knowledge.

I owe special thanks to publisher Holly L. Schmidt for her faith in me and to editor Donna Raskin for her hard work, insight, and endless encouragement. I also thank copyeditor Kristna Evans for her keen eye and long hours, and everyone else at Fair Winds for their dedication.

The following experts generously gave their time answering questions for this project:

Cynthia Sass, R.D. (nutritionist), Milly Kimball, R.D., Bonne Marano (fitness expert), Bruce Nadler, M.D. (cosmetic surgeon), Mary Lupo, M.D. (dermatologist), Claudia Kaneb (TV wardrobe chief), Arthur Jacknowitz, Pharm.D. (pharmacist), Susan Schiffman, Ph.D. (scent expert), Mark Rosekind, Ph.D. (sleep expert), Ralph Dauterive, M.D. (ob/gyn), Alison Moriarty Daley, M.S.N., P.N.P., and John Tsemberides (fitness expert). In addition, the American Dietetic Association, American Academy of Dermatology, American Society for Aesthetic Plastic Surgery, the National Sleep Foundation, the American Chiropractic Association, the Smell and Taste Research Foundation, and the American College of Obstetrics and Gynecology provided press resources.

I would also like to acknowledge Barbara Moss; Melinda Luntz of GLO in NYC; attorney Brian Murray; and my friend Dina DeSorbo-McMahon for their contributions. I thank my parents and family for their encouragement, and especially my supportive husband and daughter for sharing my attention while this book inhabited our lives.

[about the author]

Colleen Moriarty-Weston, M.S., is a freelance writer living in
Connecticut. She has a master's degree in journalism from Columbia
University Graduate School of Journalism and has been published in
several national magazines, including *Shape*, *Self*, and *Marie Claire*.
She is a contributing writer to *Fit Pregnancy* magazine.